Endovascular Neuro

Springer
*London
Berlin
Heidelberg
New York
Barcelona
Hong Kong
Milan
Paris
Santa Clara
Singapore
Tokyo*

Paul Butler (Ed.)

Endovascular Neurosurgery

A Multidisciplinary Approach

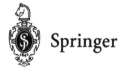

Paul Butler, MRCP, FRCR
Consultant Neuroradiologist
Department of Neuroradiology, The Royal London Hospital,
Whitechapel, London E1 1BB, UK

ISBN 978-1-84996-890-4

British Library Cataloguing in Publication Data
Endovascular neurosurgery : a multidisciplinary approach
    1. Nervous system – Surgery   2. Blood-vessels – Endoscopic
surgery
    I. Butler, Paul, 1952–
    617.4'8

Library of Congress Cataloging-in-Publication Data
Endovascular neurosurgery : a multidisciplinary approach / Paul Butler
(ed.).
        p.   cm.
    Includes bibliographical references and index.

    1. Nervous system–Surgery. 2. Blood-vessels–Endoscopic surgery.
    3. Cerebrovascular disease–Surgery. I. Butler, Paul, 1952 June 4–
    [DNLM: 1. Cerebrovascular Disorders–surgery. 2. Neurosurgical
Procedures. 3. Vascular Surgical Procedures. WL 355 E586 1999]
    RD594.2.E54   1999
    617.4'8–dc21
    DNLM/DLC
    for Library of Congress   99-32914

Apart from any fair dealing for the purposes of research or private study, or criticism or review, as permitted under the Copyright, Designs and Patents Act 1988, this publication may only be reproduced, stored or transmitted, in any form or by any means, with the prior permission in writing of the publishers, or in the case of reprographic reproduction in accordance with the terms of licences issued by the Copyright Licensing Agency. Enquiries concerning reproduction outside those terms should be sent to the publishers.

© Springer-Verlag London Limited 2010

The use of registered names, trademarks, etc. in this publication does not imply, even in ·the absence of a specific statement, that such names are exempt from the relevant laws and regulations and therefore free for general use.

Product liability: The publisher can give no guarantee for information about drug dosage and application thereof contained in this book. In every individual case the respective user must check its accuracy by consulting other pharmaceutical literature.

Preface

With a few notable exceptions, neuroradiologists have taken the lead in developing the specialty of endovascular neurosurgery. As a result they had to play a prominent role in the overall care of the patient and the patient's family, reacquainting themselves with some of the principles of the medical management of neurosurgical patients, neurological intensive care and neuroanaesthesia.

Since neuroradiologists are not primarily clinicians, from the outset there has had to be a collaboration with clinical neuroscientists, radiation therapists and anaesthetists. In my own centre, and I am sure in most others, each patient is discussed by a number of relevant specialists at specially convened meetings and a treatment plan agreed, which is then put to the patient. The neuroradiologist must be closely involved in obtaining informed consent, seeing the patient on the ward and be available subsequently, if necessary, to explain adverse outcomes to the patients and their relatives. This is a little removed from the ways of diagnostic neuroradiology, which the vast majority of neuroradiologists in the United Kingdom still practise alongside their interventional work.

Endovascular neurosurgery or interventional vascular neuroradiology is a rapidly evolving specialty and it seems that never a month passes without news of some technical innovation originating either from the manufacturing companies or from the inventive minds of neurointerventionists worldwide. This can sit a little uneasily with the current requirement for evidence-based medicine. Put simply, it is very likely, given the pace of change, that a carefully controlled study of one or other technical aspect of treatment may be overtaken by events and the information derived may thus be rendered obsolete. Additionally, many reports in the literature deal with small numbers of patients, are frequently anecdotal and may draw contradictory conclusions. Among the few large trials, the CAVATAS trial on carotid angioplasty coordinated by Atkinson Morley's and St George's Hospitals, London has proved extremely valuable. The results of the International Subarachnoid Haemorrhage Trial (ISAT) organised by the Oxford group are eagerly awaited.

Because of a perceived imperative to treat, studies on the natural history of haemorrhagic cerebrovascular disease are few and were often written decades ago. The decision to treat a lesion expectantly may be a difficult one.

This book emphasises the multidisciplinary nature of endovascular neurosurgery. The contributors have together analysed published data on the natural history of cerebral aneurysms, arteriovenous malformations and cervical arterial degenerative disease and treatment outcomes. The methodology of endovascular treatment and patient monitoring are also described and this book represents what I believe to be a balanced account of the current practice and place of endovascular neurosurgery in the United Kingdom.

Paul Butler
London 1999

Contents

1 Natural History of Intracranial Aneurysms and Vascular Malformations: Indications for Combined Surgical/Endovascular Treatment
  John S. Norris and Peter J. Hamlyn 1

2 Interventional Neuroradiology: Techniques in Embolisation of Cerebral Aneurysms and Arteriovenous Malformations
  Anil R. Gholkar and Joti J. Bhattacharya 19

3 Endovascular Treatment of Intracranial Aneurysms: The Oxford Experience
  W.E.H. Lim and James V. Byrne 39

4 Cavernous Sinus Lesions
  Robert J. Sellar 57

5 Cerebral Arteriovenous Malformations
  Robert J. Sellar 73

6 The Endovascular Treatment of Spinal Vascular Abnormalities
  Brian E. Kendall 97

7 The Endovascular Treatment of Carotid and Vertebral Artery Atherosclerotic Disease
  Andrew Clifton and Martin M. Brown 105

8 Neurological Monitoring During Endovascular Procedures
  Steven White and Richard Langford 119

9 Radiation Therapy and Vascular Malformations
  Piers N. Plowman 139

Index 157

Contributors

Joti J. Bhattacharya, MRCP, FRCR
Consultant Neuroradiologist
Institute of Neurological Sciences
Southern General Hospital
Glasgow GS1 4TF, UK

Martin M. Brown, MAMD, FRCP
Professor of Neurology
Department of Clinical Neurology
The National Hospital for Neurology
  and Neurosurgery
Queen Square
London WC1N 3BG, UK

James V. Byrne, MD, FRCS, FRCR
Consultant Neuroradiologist
Department of Neuroradiology
The Radcliffe Infirmary
Woodstock Road
Oxford OX2 6HE, UK

Andrew Clifton, MA, MRCP, FRCR
Consultant Neuroradiologist
Atkinson Morley's Hospital
Copse Hill, Wimbledon
London SW20 0RE, UK

Anil R. Gholkar, FRCR
Consultant Neuroradiologist
Newcastle General Hospital
Westgate Road
Newcastle-upon-Tyne NE4 6BE, UK

Peter J. Hamlyn, BSc, MD, FRCS, FISM
Consultant Neurosurgeon
The Royal Hospitals NHS Trust
Whitechapel, London E1 1BB, UK

Brian E. Kendall, FRCS, FRCP, FRCR
Consultant Neuroradiologist
The Royal Free Hospital
Pond Street
London NW3 2QG, UK

Richard Langford, FRCA
Senior Lecturer and Hon. Consultant Anaesthetist
St Bartholomew's Hospital
38 Little Britain
West Smithfield
London EC1A 7BE, UK

W.E.H. Lim, FRCR
Consultant Radiologist
Singapore General Hospital
Outram Road
Singapore 0316

John S. Norris, FRCS (SN)
Consultant Neurosurgeon
Hurstwood Park Neurological Centre
The Princess Royal Hospital
Haywards Heath
West Sussex RH16 4EX, Uk

Piers N. Plowman, MA, MD, FRCP, FRCR
Consultant Radiotherapist
St Bartholomew's Hospital
38 Little Britain
West Smithfield
London EC1A 7BE, UK

Robert J. Sellar, MRCP, FRCR
Consultant Neuroradiologist
Western General Hospital
Crewe Road South
Edinburgh EH4 2XU, UK

Steven White, DPhil, MRCPsych
Consultant Neurophysiologist
St Bartholomew's Hospital
38 Little Britain
West Smithfield
London EC1A 7BE, UK

Chapter 1
Natural History of Intracranial Aneurysms and Vascular Malformations: Indications for Combined Surgical/Endovascular Treatment

John S. Norris and Peter J. Hamlyn

Natural History

The natural history of intracranial aneurysms and arteriovenous malformations is difficult to determine accurately, because those presenting with haemorrhage usually require surgical treatment. The majority of those who have not bled are not discovered, although this may change with the wider availability of magnetic resonance imaging and magnetic resonance angiography.

Intracranial arterial aneurysms, arteriovenous malformations and other vascular anomalies are relatively rare in the population but, when they are present, they have the potential to cause morbidity and death. An appreciation of the natural history of these conditions is important as the morbidity and mortality of treatment has improved considerably. In most, the treatment now carries less risk than the natural history of the lesion once haemorhage has occurred. Earlier or late surgery for those who are fit enough provides better outcomes and lower mortality than conservative treatment (Heros et al., 1990; Saveland et al., 1992). Incidentally discovered lesions may also be offered treatment electively to forestall the development of symptoms, though the statistics have been less compelling.

Saccular Aneurysms

These so-called "berry" aneurysms arise at points of congenital weakness in the arterial wall. They are found in all age groups but become increasingly common with age (Pakarinen, 1967).

Ruptured Saccular Aneurysms

For many years it has been known that an aneurysm which has ruptured once has a high risk of rupturing again. It was reported in the 1950s that, without treatment

20% of patients would remain well, 20% would be disabled and 60% would die eventually from either the initial or a subsequent ictus (Ask-Upmark & Ingvar, 1950). Further studies (Joensen, 1984) have confirmed this.

In an analysis of 589 cases Pakarinen (Pakarinen, 1967) found that, within a defined population, 43%, (including those who did not reach hospital), died as a result of the initial haemorrhage and that by the end of the first and fifth years, the mortality had increased to 63% and 72%, respectively. Seventy-four per cent of deaths occurred within the first 24 hours of the initial bleed with 14% dying prior to arriving in hospital. In this study only 91 (15.5%) had surgery. This study gives a reasonable appreciation of the natural history of the untreated ruptured aneurysms.

One of the early co-operative studies (Sahs et al., 1969) reported that 20% of deaths occurred in the first 48 hours (excluding those dying before reaching hospital), 40% within the first week and 67% within the first 3 weeks. Bleeding from anterior circulation aneurysms was greater during the earlier period, being 10% in the first week, 12% in the second week, 6.9% in the third week, 8.2% in the fourth week and 1.3% per week for the next eight weeks. The rate of rebleeding peaked at 4% per day on day 7, being greatest for anterior communicating artery aneurysms and lowest for middle cerebral artery aneurysms. A more recent collaborative study (Kassell & Torner, 1983) demonstrated a peak incidence of rebleeding within the first 24 hours (4%). The rate of rebleeding dropped sharply until the end of the second day, when it was approximately 1.5% per day and it declined thereafter for the duration of the study period. The cumulative rebleeding rate was 19% at 14 days.

Patients with untreated ruptured aneurysms continue to have a substantial long-term risk. In a late follow up of 568 patients treated conservatively (Nishioka et al., 1984) in a co-operative study, reported that the rate of rebleeding after 6 months was 2.2% per year for the first 9.5 years and 0.86% per year for the subsequent decade. Alvord (Alvord et al., 1972) used the data from Pakarinen's (Pakarinen, 1967) and McKissock's (McKissock et al., 1965) published data to construct a table accurately estimating survival up to 10 years following haemorrhage. It was based on only two clinical observations: the duration of survival from the first or most recent haemorrhage and the clinical grading of patient at the time of assessment. They also confirmed that the highest risk of further haemorrhage is during the first 2 weeks after the initial event.

Unruptured Saccular Aneurysms

Unruptured aneurysms may be classified by their size, multiplicity and whether or not they are symptomatic. They are most likely to be discovered during conventional or magnetic resonance (MR) angiography for the investigation of haemorrhage from another aneurysm or vascular malformation. Larger aneurysms can be discovered serendipitously during scanning for a variety of unrelated reasons. Magnetic resonance angiography is being used increasingly to screen patients with suspicious headache or with a family history of intracranial haemorrhage.

In a follow up (4 months to 11 years) study of 76 patients with haemorrhage and multiple aneurysms, in whom unruptured aneurysms were not treated, Heiskanen (Heiskanen, 1970) found that 8 (10.5%) of the incidental aneurysms bled, 3 (4%) fatally (Table 1.1). In a later study of 61 patients with subarachnoid haemorrhage and multiple aneurysms followed from 10 to 24 years (including some from the previous study), the same group (Heiskanen, 1981) reported that 16% of the patients bled from previously unruptured aneurysms, with a 57% mortality rate.

Table 1.1. Natural history of unruptured aneurysms

Reference	Number of changes	Number of haemorrhages	%	Follow-up
Moyes, 1971	29	4	13	1–10 years
Heiskanen, 1970	76	8	10	0.5–11 years
Heiskanen, 1981	61	10	16	16 years
Wiebers et al. 1987	130	15	11	8.3 years

Winn et al. (1983) assessed 182 patients with subarachnoid haemorrhage and multiple aneurysms that were followed for an average of 8 years. Fifty patients underwent craniotomy to clip the ruptured aneurysms whilst the remaining 132 were treated with bed rest. Thirty per cent of the latter group rebled with an average annual rebleeding rate of 3%. It was always the previously ruptured aneurysms that caused the rebleed. In the 38 patients who survived surgery for clipping of a ruptured aneurysm, the smallest risk of rupture of the untreated asymptomatic aneurysms was 1% per year. The minimum risk of the asymptomatic aneurysm rupturing during the remaining lifetime has been calculated (Table 1.2) (Dell, 1982).

Giant aneurysms are, by definition, greater than 2.5 cm in diameter. They have a dismal prognosis, with up to 80% dying from rupture or compression of vital structures (Sonntag et al., 1977). There are isolated reports of giant aneurysms diminishing in size or even disappearing completely (Scott & Ballatine, 1972). The risk of rupture is highest in symptomatic aneurysms and that risk increases with size (Redekop & Ferguson, 1995).

Recent retrospective data from an ongoing prospective series at the Mayo clinic (Wiebers, 1998) found that the risk of an unruptured aneurysm of less than 10 mm diameter, rupturing was 0.05% p.a. Those patients with previous subarachnoid haemorrhage harbouring unruptured aneurysm had an annual haemorrhage rate, from the unruptured aneurysm, 11 times higher (0.5% p.a.). Overall, the surgical risks of surgery in unruptured aneurysms less than 10 mm were far greater than the 7.5-year-risk. More information will become available at a later date.

Table 1.2. Risks of rupture of incidental, asymptomatic aneurysms during the remaining life span (Dell, 1982)

Age presenting (years)	Risk of haemorrhage (%)
20	16.6
30	16.1
40	14.4
50	10.3
60	4.7

Surgery: Indications

Ruptured Saccular Aneurysms

With the high risk of rebleeding, the decision to operate must be balanced against the risks of surgery to the brain. The timing of surgery has been the subject of much study. It can be classified thus:

- Early surgery occurs within 72 hours of aneurysmal rupture.
- Intermediate surgery takes place between 4 and 10 days.
- Thereafter surgery is regarded as "delayed".

In the 1970s and 1980s most surgeons practised delayed surgery. Using this policy, the Danish Aneurysm Study Group (Rosenorn et al., 1987) reported an overall normal outcome of 27% and a mortality rate of 45.5% in 1076 patients, who were alive on admission to hospital. Subsequently, a prospective randomised study (Ohman & Heiskanen 1989) was carried out encompassing 216 patients in clinical Hunt & Hess grades I to III.

Numerous clinical grading systems for subarachnoid haemorrhage are available. Four are in common use, with the Hunt & Hess being one of the more frequently encountered in the 1970s and 1980s. In 1988 the World Federation of Neurosurgeons (WFNS) proposed a simpler and more intuitive five-point grading systems, which is being increasingly used as it is based on the objective criteria of the Glasgow Coma Score and the presence/absence of the neurological deficits.

Surgery within 3 days following haemorrhage was not found to be associated with higher morbidity or mortality rates. The outcome at 3 months following haemorrhage was associated with marginally better results compared with the intermediate and late groups. More recent prospective studies (Saveland et al., 1992) have again demonstrated patients in good clinical condition, operated on early, have a mortality of between 20 and 25% and good recovery in 55 to 65%. Others (Kassell et al., 1990) only demonstrate benefit in patients operated on early or late. Overall, those in the intermediate group do worse.

These studies provide good evidence to suggest that there is substantial benefit to be gained from early, or even ultra-early, surgery if there is space-occupying intracerebral haemorrhage, with aggressive management of cerebral ischaemia (should it arise) following rupture of intracranial aneurysms.

Unruptured Saccular Aneurysms

Although the risks of surgery to exclude these aneurysms from the circulation are less than if they had ruptured (Saveland et al., 1992), the risks are real and careful counselling of the patient and family regarding the risks and benefits of surgery needs to take place.

The size, shape and location of the aneurysm itself influence the outcome. Aneurysms less than 3 mm in diameter may be difficult to clip surgically and those larger than 10 mm are likely to rupture and some believe they should be excluded from the circulation if this is safe (Cromwell et al., 1995). If the lesion is greater than 15 mm in diameter, the risk of surgical correction may be greater (Wirth et al., 1983; Wirth, 1986) than leaving the aneurysms untreated. Giant aneurysms (greater than 25 mm diameter) have even more risk associated with treatment, although some groups have published excellent surgical results (Heiskanen, 1986).

The location of the aneurysm is an important factor. Internal carotid aneurysms are more favourable to treat (Wirth et al., 1983; Wirth, 1986). Aneurysms with wide necks are more demanding to obliterate successfully either by direct surgery or endovascular coiling. A calcified sac indicates poor compliance, restricting access for the surgeon and so increasing the risk of distorting the surrounding anatomical structures. While no scientific data exist to allow these factors to be quantified, they should clearly influence the decision to operate.

Patient-related factors have a bearing on the likely outcome of treatment. Age is of paramount importance. The younger the patient, the greater the risk of eventual rupture of incidental aneurysms as the annual risks become cumulative (Table 1.2). Serious medical conditions such as neoplasia and cerebral vascular disease will act to shorten life expectancy, making neurosurgical intervention an unnecessary threat to an already foreshortened life.

Incidental aneurysms found during pregnancy are best followed non-operatively until after delivery, unless concern arises that imminent rupture is due or a difficult labour likely (Crowell et al., 1995). Intuitively it would be advisable for delivery to be by elective Caesarean section avoiding uncontrollable Valsalva manoeuvres with consequent wide fluctuations of blood pressure and intracranial pressure.

The following recommendations have been proposed by experienced groups (Cromwell et al., 1995).

1. Those aneurysms associated with symptoms are at significant risk of rupture and treatment is generally warranted.
2. Familial aneurysms can rupture regardless of size and treatment is therefore usually justified.
3. Multiple unruptured aneurysms may bleed even if small (6–9 mm) and again treatment is often warranted.
4. The risk of truly incidental aneurysms rupturing depends on size.

Aneurysms less than 7 millimetres diameter have a low risk of haemorrhage and so careful follow up is recommended. In cases of increasing size, treatment should be offered.

Aneurysms of 10 mm and greater threaten to haemorrhage, so treatment is usually indicated.

Aneurysms between 7 and 10 mm in diameter are in an ill-defined group, may be managed conservatively or actively depending on the general health and age of the patient and the location of the aneurysm.

5. Microsurgical occlusion is very successful and is the treatment of choice. The best anatomical features are diameters of between 3 and 15 mm, narrow necks, minimal or no calcification, non-adherent perforating branches and internal carotid, middle cerebral or even anterior communicating artery locations. Peroperative angiography is of great benefit for proximal internal carotid aneurysms.
6. Guglielmi detachable coil (GDC) treatment can be used with low risk and successful obliteration in most cases. Treatment may be safer when the risks of surgery are high, where the aneurysms diameter is greater than 15 mm, basilar or anterior communicating artery aneurysms, calcification or adherent perforator branches. Diameters of less than 5 mm and broad necks are relative contraindications. An experienced radiologist is a prerequisite.
7. Sometimes, incidental aneurysms that are not suitable for clip or coil treatment may be candidates for surgical or balloon occlusion of the parent vessel with distal bypass.

Non-saccular intracranial aneurysms

Fusiform Aneurysms

Fusiform aneurysms tend to occur on vessels as a result of atherosclerotic loss of elasticity or other trauma (e.g. radiotherapy). Up to 80% are found on the vertebrobasilar circulation (Goldstein & Tibbs 1981)

The natural history of these lesions is not well known, but they typically present with cranial nerve or brain stem compression and rarely manifest with haemorrhage or thrombosis.

Traumatic Aneurysms

Traumatic aneurysms occur as a result of injury to the arterial wall and they are usually false, with rupture of the three layers of the vessel wall. Fibrous organisation of the haematoma leads to formation of an aneurysm. They tend to be located on the longitudinal aspect of the arterial wall as compared to saccular aneurysms, which mainly occur at bifurcations. They occur only rarely in the posterior circulation and are usually located on the middle or anterior cerebral arteries (Fleischer et al., 1975).

The natural history is variable. A review (Fleischer et al., 1975) of 41 cases following penetrating and blunt head injuries, has shown an overall mortality of 27% with an 18% mortality for those treated surgically and 41% mortality in those treated conservatively, with over half rupturing within 3 weeks of the initial injury. However, no account was taken of the severity or sequelae of the initial cerebral injury. Seventeen (43%) had presented with delayed subarachnoid haemorrhage following head injury with time intervals ranging from 2 days to 6 weeks.

Infective (Mycotic) Aneurysms

The majority of these aneurysms arise at the sites of microemboli from cardiac or pulmonary sepsis. However, cardiac surgery, renal dialysis and intravenous drug abuse are increasingly common causes. Bacteria or fungi are known to be the causative agents. Damage to the intima and loss of elastic tissue due to focal inflammatory tissue are the characteristic pathologies. The weakened vessel wall dilates to form an aneurysm encased by inflammatory tissue. These lesions are most commonly found in cases of endocarditis, with large ragged vegetations on the cardiac valve leaflets (Weir, 1987). Reviews have been published (Ojeman, 1985), based on experience gained from 81 patients found to have infective aneurysms having developed symptoms and then having undergone cerebral angiography.

Of 30 treated with antibiotics alone, 13 died. Twenty-nine patients underwent surgery with two fatalities due to rupture from haemorrhage from other initially occult infective aneurysms. The authors recommend that haemorrhage from a distal middle cerebral artery aneurysm should be treated by excision of the aneurysm and sacrifice of the vessel, providing the patient is fit for surgery. Those aneurysms on proximal vessels, unruptured aneurysms or those in locations where the sacrifice of the vessel would not be tolerated should be treated conservatively with antibiotics and serial angiography at fortnightly intervals. Infective aneurysms, which persist or enlarge, should be operated upon.

It is increasingly felt that infective aneurysms are unstable, unpredictable and, regardless of dimension, prone to rupture with all the consequences of morbidity and mortality (Holtzman et al., 1995). One group (Holtzman et al., 1995) has reviewed the literature and their own experience, concluding with the recommendation that single accessible infected aneurysms in medically stable patients should be promptly excised.

Direct clip application is always difficult due to the friable inflammatory sac. It may be more appropriate to occlude the parent vessel and/or trap the aneurysm at the risk of neurological deficit. Endovascular treatment is increasingly being used as experience accumulates (Holtzman et al., 1995).

Vascular Malformations

Most intracranial vascular anomalies are congenital, but they may enlarge over time. Arteriovenous malformations are the most likely to require intervention and are therefore discussed first, with mention of particular situations such as presentation in childhood or during pregnancy.

Dural arteriovenous malformations form a separate subgroup, although they remain in essence a shunt of arterial blood to the venous circulation without an intervening capillary bed.

Venous angiomas occur in a familial and sporadic forms, causing significant morbidity, but are less common than arteriovenous malformations. However, they are increasingly reported on MRI. Venous angiomas are one of the commonest anomalies found at post mortem (Sarwar & McCormick 1978) but are usually silent clinically.

Arteriovenous Malformations

Arteriovenous malformations are developmental anomalies of the intracranial vasculature, which may progress throughout the lifetime of a patient. They have a haemorrhage rate of 1–2.3% per annum (whether the lesion has bled or not) quoted in textbooks (Garretson, 1985). The primary pathological lesion consists of one or more persisting connections between the arterial inflow and the venous outflow without an intervening capillary bed. The most recent estimates from post-mortem studies of the prevalence of all types of cerebral vascular malformation are around 4.7% and, for arteriovenous malformations, 0.5% (McCormick, 1984).

The co-operative study on intracranial aneurysms and arteriovenous malformations suggests that the frequency of the latter is one seventh that of saccular aneurysms (Perret & Nishioka 1966). The majority of arteriovenous malformations become symptomatic by the age of 40 years and there is a slight male preponderance (Wilkins, 1985).

Decision making for treatment requires knowledge and accurate information on the clinical course and natural history of these lesions (Wilkins, 1985; Heros & Tu, 1986). Knowledge of the natural history of arteriovenous malformations is imperfect because of the imperative to treat a substantial proportion of cases which results in a selection bias in those left untreated. Conservative treatment of a natural population of arteriovenous malformations is unlikely to be tolerated today, hence our reliance on studies from 20 or more years ago. Data from this period forms the basis of more recently published material from the 1980s. Furthermore, the behaviour of untreated arteriovenous malformations is not the same as the natural history of the condition, as not all arteriovenous malformation are identified and not all those found are followed for an adequate length of time without treatment.

Arteriovenous malformations present with intracranial haemorrhage in 50%, seizures in 25% and other symptoms in 25% of patients (Martin & Vinters 1996). Early bleeding after the initial ictus is rare and thus much less frequent than with intracranial aneurysms. Graf et al. (1983) estimate the risk of symptomatic AVM haemorrhage is 6% during the first year, while Fults and Kelly (1984) state that it is as high as 17%. The risks of haemorrhage tend to be evenly distributed through the first year (Perret & Nishioka 1966).

The long-term risk of rebleeding after the first haemorrhage has been assessed by several authors, (Forster et al., 1972; Graf et al., 1983; Fults & Kelly 1984; Torner, 1985; Crawford et al., 1986; Ondra et al., 1990). These show a fairly consistent rate of between 2 and 3% per annum. Ondra's group (Ondra et al., 1990) followed prospectively the conservative treatment of arteriovenous malformations in 166 patients and quote a haemorrhage rate of 4% per year, with a mortality rate of 1% per year. The mean interval between initial presentation and further haemorrhage was 7.7 years.

The rate of rebleeding appears to increase in patients who have had more than one haemorrhage. Forster et al. (1972) found that, following the initial bleed, there was one in four chance of bleeding again in 4 years. A patient suffering two haemorrhages has a one in four chance of a third in the next 12 months. Crawford et al., (1986) state that there is a 40% risk of rebleeding within 15 years in patients following the initial episode and 58% risk in those who have experienced multiple episodes. Some studies find the risk of haemorrhage reduces after 15 to 20 years (Fults & Kelly 1984; Ondra et al., 1990).

The risk of neurological deficit after a haemorrhage is between 30% (Samson & Baljer 1991) and 50% (Wilkins, 1985). Fults and Kelly found that, of patients with arteriovenous malformations presenting with a first haemorrhage, 13.6% died from that haemorrhage, 20.7% from the second and 25% from the third. (Fults & Kelly, 1984) After the first haemorrhage the chance of patient going on to develop a further haemorrhage was 67.4% with an overall risk death from haemorrhage of 40.5%.

Unruptured arteriovenous malformations, which have not bled, have only slightly less risk of rupturing than those who have bled previously (Table 1.3), excluding the initial high rate of rupture in the first year after haemorrhage. Generally the rate is quoted to be in the region of 2–3% per annum (Brown et al., 1988; Forster et al., 1972; Graf et al., 1983; Fults & Kelly, 1984; Torner, 1985; Crawford et al., 1986; Ondra et al., 1990;). Asymptomatic lesions have the same risk of haemorrhage as those presenting with seizures or neurological deficit.

Prospective series' following the conservative treatment of arteriovenous malformations are rare but Ondra's group (Ondra et al., 1990) did this in a Finnish popu-

Table 1.3. Risks of haemorrhage, morbidity and mortality from unrupted (and ruptured) AVMs (Morcos, 1995)

Reference	Average annual rates of				
	No of cases	Bleeding (%)	Morbidity (%)	Mortality (%)	Average years of follow-up
Perret & Nishioka, 1966	77	1.5	–	–	20
Kelly et al., 1969	26	–	2.8	0.9	12.5
Forster et al., 1972	46	1.7	1.3	1.1	15
Graf et al., 1983	71	2	–	–	20
Fults & Kelly, 1984	26	3	2.2	1.3	8.7
Brown et al., 1988	168	2.2	2.8	0.7	8.2
Crawford et al., 1986	77 (140)*	1.7 (2.6)*	1 (1)*	1.5 (1.6)*	10.4
Ondra et al., 1990	46 (114)*	4.2 (3.9)*	0.7 (2.4)*	0.9 (1)*	23.7

* Bracketted figures apply to ruptured AVMs.
AVM, arteriovenous malformation.

lation. One hundred and sixty-six patients, who were not treated surgically, were followed prospectively for an average of 20 years. Twenty-three died from haemorrhage with a 2.7% per annum combined mortality and morbidity rate. The annual rate of morbidity however was substantially higher for patients who were presented initially with haemorrhage, presumably due to the cumulative effect of neutral damage. The mean age of death in the cohort from all causes was 51 years (the average life span was 73 years in the normal Finnish population at that time).

Arteriovenous malformations are dynamic lessions and are known to have a propensity to enlarge with time if untreated. There is evidence to suggest that patients below 30 years of age are most at risk of this enlargement (Menedelow et al., 1987). Children and young adults should be considered candidates for definitive treatment to minimise the risk of morbidity and mortality with the passage of time as nearly one hundred per cent of children who have bled from an arteriovenous malformation will do so again within 10 years (Manelfe et al., 1990).

The risk of a patient having a seizure after bleeding from an arteriovenous malformation is about 1% per year. In the co-operative study, 28% of patients with supratentorial arteriovenous malformations had seizures (Perret et al., 1966) with 25% experiencing a seizure prior to the haemorrhage of supratentorial lesions. Fults and Kelly (Fults & Kelly 1984) stated that a patient with an arteriovenous malformation presenting with seizures alone has a 26% chance of suffering a haemorrhage and an 11.6% chance of dying from the event.

Medically intractable epilepsy, secondary to an unruptured arteriovenous malformation may be an indication for surgical intervention. The indications for surgery are not as clear as when an arteriovenous malformation presents with haemorrhage in addition to seizures.

The decision to treat surgically will depend on the severity and frequency of the convulsions and the location and size of the arteriovenous malformation. Ligation or embolisation of arteriovenous malformation feeders results in cure of seizures in 18% of cases, whilst complete surgical excision of the nidus and the abnormal vessels increases this to approximately 56%. Sometimes the epileptogenic focus is also in the adjacent cortex. In very select cases, cortical excision of these areas can increase the cure rate to 75% (Weinand, 1996).

Arteriovenous Malformations in Pregnancy

Intracranial haemorrhage from aneurysms and arteriovenous malformations is equal during pregnancy, giving the impression that pregnancy increases the risk of haemorrhage from an arteriovenous malformation. Horton et al. (1990) studied retrospectively a total of 540 pregnancies in 451 women. Seventeen pregnancies were complicated by intracranial haemorrhage. They found that the haemorrhage rate during pregnancy for women with unruptured arteriovenous malformations were 3.5% and for non-pregnant women of child-bearing age from the same entity 3.1%. This suggests that pregnancy for women harbouring an arteriovenous malformation does not constitute a significant risk factor.

Robinson et al. (1974) presented 11 patients whose arteriovenous malformations had bled during pregnancy and of these, three had recurrent haemorrhage during the same pregnancy. However Ondra presented to the American Association of Neurosurgeons (AANS) in 1992 a study based on his 166 Finnish patients with arteriovenous malformations published previously (Ondra et al., 1990). The studies found that 14% of all haemorrhages occurred in the last trimester of pregnancy or immediately post-partum and suggested those women harbouring symptomatic arteriovenous malformations during pregnancy are at greater risk of rupture. Significantly, in both series, no rupture occurred during that actual birth (labour or caesarean section), but as with aneurysms, it would seem prudent to undertake an elective caesarean section. Others (Martin & Wilson, 1984) have reported successful outcomes to operating on vascular malformation during pregnancy, with the large majority doing well.

There is currently no accurate risk assessment of arteriovenous malformation rupture during pregnancy. Overall, the other evidence suggests that a pregnant woman presenting with haemorrhage or increasing neurological deficit from arteriovenous malformation should be considered for immediate surgical excision.

Childhood Arteriovenous Malformations

The prognosis for untreated arteriovenous malformation in children appears to be worse than in adults (Sedzmir & Robinson, 1973; Mori et al., 1980; Gerosa et al., 1981; Senegor et al., 1983; Celli et al., 1984). The probability of bleeding after the first clinical presentation was approximately 5% per annum. Some results suggest that the risk of haemorrhage is higher in the paediatric population than in adults (Celli et al., 1984). In addition, the annual rate of mortality related to younger patients of less than 15 years was greater than 2% compared with 1.5% in adults. Fults and Kelly (1984) reported on eight children managed conservatively for around 8 years and only three remaining well. Three died and two became disabled.

Dural Arteriovenous Malformations

Dural arteriovenous malformations are mainly encountered above the age of 40 years in both sexes (Luessenhop, 1985). Information on the natural history of these lesions is incomplete, with no long-term follow-up series to record the outcome of patients with this condition with any reliability, (Awad, 1996). Haemorrhage, which is usually intradural, is the most frequent complication (Malik et al., 1984; Luessenhop, 1985).

In 1990 Awad (Awad et al., 1990) presented a review of 377 dural arteriovenous malformations reported in the literature at that time. Seventeen were from their own department. Intracranial haemorrhage occurred in 88 (23%), non-haemorrhagic focal neurological deficit in 12 (3%) and no focal deficits or haemorrhage (seizures, headaches, etc.) in 277 (73.5%). Serious neurological symptoms correlated with retrograde leptomeningeal venous drainage, variceal or aneurysmal venous structures and deep venous drainage. No correlation was found with the site of the lesion or the rate of shunting despite a clear association of haemorrhage with dural arteriovenous malformations in certain locations. The report concludes that (retrograde) leptomeningeal venous drainage is an ominous feature for dural arteriovenous malformation in whatever location and it specifically predisposes these lesions to intracranial haemorrhage or other serious neurological sequelae. Even non-haemorrhagic focal deficits were associated with leptomeningeal venous engorgement. The initial haemorrhage is associated with a mortality of 30% but those on anticoagulants this is much higher and consequently anticoagulation is specifically contraindicated in those with evidence of retrograde leptomeningeal venous drainage.

The classification describes by Borden et al. (1995) identifies three types of dural asteriovenous malformation:

1. Simple shunting within the dural leaflets, patent venous sinuses and no reflux in to the leptomeningeal (cortical veins).
2. Some of the blood shunted through the fistula discharges into a (usually partly occluded) venous sinus *and* into the leptomeningeal veins, which are engorged.
3. Occluded venous sinus, with all blood shunted through the fistula draining only into the leptomeningeal veins.

Davies et al. (1996) has validated this classification with the type of presentation and adverse neurological events. He went on to confirm (Davies et al., 1997a) that Borden 1 lesions have a benign natural history, with 53 of 54 patients (98%), prospectively followed over 11 years, not experiencing adverse neurological events. Borden II & III lesion are associated with "aggressive" behaviour (Davies et al., 1997b). Fourteen patients selected conservative treatment over the 11-year period (249 lesion months). During follow- up four (29%) died and, excluding presentation, these patients were observed to have interval rates of intracranial haemorrhage, non-haemorrhagic neurological deficit and mortality of 19.2%, 10.9% and 19.3% per lesion year, respectively. The persistence of retrograde leptomeningeal venous drainage after treatment was also associated with poor outcome.

Cases of haemorrhage where there is no leptomeningeal venous drainage exist but are very rare (Awad, 1990). The actual risk of haemorrhage in this group is unknown (Awad, 1996).

Other large studies concur with Awad's contention that lesions adjacent to widely patent venous sinuses are less likely to develop leptomeningeal venous drainage than those lesions with compromised dural venous drainage (Malik et al., 1984; Lasjaunias et al., 1986). Specifically lesions at the incisura and the other anterior cranial fossa are rarely found without leptomeningeal venous drainage. However, those around the cavernous and transverse sinuses rarely show this pattern of venous drainage unless there is venous outflow obstruction. It is known what predisposes a particular lesion to progress, to develop leptomeningeal venous drainage or to resolve spontaneously (Awad, 1996).

Cavernous Haemangiomas

Cavernous haemangiomas constitute 8 to 15% of intracranial vascular malformations and occur in 0.1 to 0.5% of the general population (Wascher & Spetzler, 1995). There is a familial and a sporadic form. The former has a more aggressive natural history with a 6.5% per patient, per annum or 1.3% per annum per lesion risk of further haemorrhage following the initial bleed and neurological deterioration occurring at a rate of 15% per annum. The risk of further haemorrhage from the sporadic type is approximately 0.25 to 0.7% per annum (Wascher & Spetzler 1995).

Nevertheless, cavernous haemangiomas are mainly asymptomatic lesions found coincidentally on computed tarography (CT), MRI or at post mortem. They are found at all ages with an equal sex incidence. Seventy-six percent are supratentorial (Voigt & Yasargil 1976). Characteristically, angiography fails to delineate what appears to be a discrete lesion on CT or MRI. There is not a typical presentation but the acute or subacute onset of headache, fits and neurological deficits (intracerebral or subarachnoid haemorrhage) may occur. In one series (Giombini & Morello, 1978), 51 symptomatic lesions (including 37 from the literature) were reviewed.

Twelve (24%) presented with intracranial haemorrhage, which was rapidly fatal in three (1.5%) and 19 (37%) with seizures. Five underwent surgery after the first haemorrhage. In the remaining group, two had a further fatal bleed, after asymptomatic intervals of 2 and 7 years, respectively. A third patient had a further haemorrhage after 10 asymptomatic years, with a fourth bleeding 9 and 12 months after the initial haemorrhage. These patients were cured by surgery to remove the lesion.

The Toronto Vascular Malformation Study Group (Porter et al., 1997) presented the prospectively collected data on 173 patients harbouring one or more cavernomas. The mean age of presentation was 37.5 years. There were 18 interval events in 427 patient years of follow-up, for an overall annual event rate of 4.2%. Location of the lesions was the most important predictive factor of neurological events: 10.6% per year in "deep" and 0% per year for "superficial" lesions.

Our knowledge of these lesions remains incomplete and contentious issues remain regarding management, (Sparrow, 1998). The relative indications for surgery are to establish a tissue diagnosis, remove mass effect causing deficit or seizures and to remove or prevent intracranial haematomas.

Venous Angiomas

These are among the most frequently encountered intracranial vascular malformations found at autopsy, occurring in 2.5% of cases (Sarwar & McCormick, 1978) with the majority remaining asymptomatic throughout life. They are predominantly silent clinically, seldom causing symptoms, but increasingly frequently turning up on CT and MRI scans. They are increasingly associated with the presence of carvernous haemangiomas. Cerebral angiography reveals a characteristics "caput medusae" appearance.

In 1982 Numaguchi (Numaguchi et al., 1982) presented 61 cases (including 11 of their own). The male: female ratio was 37:24 with an age range of 9 to 63 years. Fifty-nine (96.8%) had a solitary lesion with multiple angiomas in two patients (3.2%). Seventeen (27.9%) were within the infratentorial compartment. Seizures were the main presenting symptom in 14 (23%) with eight (13%) presenting with haemorrhage.

Cerebellar venous angiomas have a greater propensity to bleed, occurring in 36%, (Rothfus et al., 1984). Therefore there should be a lower threshold to intervene in venous angiomas of the posterior fossa.

Conclusions

Precise prediction of the natural history of intracranial aneurysms and vascular malformation is based on data acquired prior to the development of microneurosurgery and endovascular neuroradiology. All may rupture and expose patients to the risk of neurological deficit and death. There is also the risk of further haemorrhage and non-haemorrhagic neurological decline.

Aneurysmal rebleeding is highest shortly after a haemorrhage, whilst arteriovenous malformations have a cumulative that is not influenced by whether haemorrhage has occurred or not, except perhaps during the first 12 months.

The co-operative (and other) studies from 30 years ago provide us with the only satisfactory data upon which to determine accurately the natural history of untreated arteriovenous malformations, aneurysms and other vascular anomalies. Long-term follow up, accurate data collection and peer review will help to ensure that the treatments for intracranial vascular abnormalities are safer options than exposure to the natural history.

Combined Surgical/Endovascular Treatment

In the multidisciplinary approach to the management of cerebral vascular lesions, treatments are tailored to the individual patient and may involve embolisation, surgery or radiotherapy, either alone or in combination. Endovascular procedures for arteriovenous malformations normally precede any surgery and are often "staged" at interval of days or weeks to gauge their effect and to exploit any progressive obliteration that may occur. There are, nevertheless, some situations where a combined simultaneous surgical and endovascular approach may be the most expeditious means of dealing safely with an aneurysm or arteriovenous malformation (Hacein-Bey et al., 1998).

The concept of endovascular treatment has its origins in neurosurgery. Dott (Dott, 1969) in 1941 in Edinburgh, was the first to describe treating aneurysms by opening the sac and inserting muscle to cause thrombosis in 1941. Gallagher (Gallagher, 1964) introduced horsehair into the aneurysmal sac to induce thrombosis. Mullan (Mullan et al., 1965) used wires and the passage of an electrical current to achieve the same effect. Guglielmi (Guglielmi et al., 1991) first reported the use in humans of the detachable platinum coils which now bear his name and which are the most commonly used form of endovascular treatment for intracranial aneurysms.

Aneurysms

The mainstay of treatment of intracranial aneurysms has long been open surgery to clip and exclude the sac from the arterial circulation (Kassell et al., 1990). Endovascular treatment of aneurysms may be required when the location of the aneurysm, its size or shape makes surgery or access technically difficult. It may also be necessary when a patient is in a poor medical condition. All of these factors significantly increase the risks of surgical intervention (Higashida et al., 1990). Trials of this as a frontline treatment are ongoing.

A combined simultaneous surgical and endovascular approach has been used to deal safely with aneurysms of the posterior circulation and of the paraclinoid carotid artery. Bailes et al. (1992) published a series of four females presenting with subarachnoid haemorrhage from basilar tip aneurysms that were dealt with successfully surgically by utilising non-detachable balloons to obtain proximal control of the basilar trunk whilst the aneurysm was dissected and manipulated. A more recent series (Mizoi et al., 1994) of five patients with basilar trunk aneurysms described no distal embolic complications or vessel or damage where the mean temporary occlusion time was 22 minutes. The same group had previously used this technique in dealing with nine paraclinoid carotid aneurysms (Mizoi et al., 1993). In six cases the sac was aspirated to collapse the aneurysm, facilitating easier placement of the clip. There was one embolic complication. Experience of these combined techniques continues to emerge (Hacien-Bey et al., 1998).

Arteriovenous Malformations

Small arteriorvenous malformations located superficially in non-eloquent areas, which have bled, are best treated by primary surgical excision (Khayata et al., 1995).

Large arteriovenous malformations, which are often near to or within, eloquent brain tissue, are usually treated by a combination of embolisation, radiosurgery and surgery and usually in that order.

Pre-operative embolisation and peroperative angiography are routinely used in some centres though the combining of open surgery with simultaneous endovascular procedures is infrequently employed. However, it appears to be valuable in selected cases. It may not be possible, for example, even with the current microcatheter systems, either to reach some arterial pedicles safely or to deliver the necessary volume of glue to the lesion. It may therefore be valuable to undertake intraoperative placement of catheters into the arterial feeders by microsurgical dissection. An aneurysm clip is placed on the proximal vessel and the distal portion is selectively catheterised with the microcatheter (Girvin et al., 1983). With a proximal artery clip in position there is almost no risk of retrograde entry of glue into normal cerebral vessels.

Khayata et al. (1995) recommended "maximum aggressive" percutaneous transfemoral endovascular treatment. Residual feeders are subsequently dealt with intraoperatively, in the manner described above and any residuum is treated with stereotactic radiosurgery. Results are encouraging with the same group reporting a mean decrease of 86% in the size of the arteriovenous malformations in 10 patients treated.

Conclusion

An inherent disadvantage of open surgical clipping of aneurysms, particularly those which are very large or which are located in the posterior circulation, is the inability to achieve proximal "control" with exposure of the aneurysmal sac. The risk of uncontrolled haemorrhage can be reduced using non-detachable balloon catheters in the parent artery.

Microsurgical dissection may be used to place microcatheters in small, otherwise inaccessible feeders to large or deeply located arteriovenous malformation and enable the delivery of larger volumes of glue to the lesion.

In these situations a combined surgical and interventional radiological approach provides the opportunity to benefit from the direct access afforded by surgery with minimal distortion of surrounding brain. In the case of aneurysms, endovascular techniques produce proximal "control", whereas with arteriovenous malformations this control is provided by microsurgery.

Whether treatments are staged or simultaneous, high quality surgical and radiological facilities need to be co-located to enhance the collaboration between neurosurgeons, radiologists and radiation therapists if these difficult conditions are to be treated most effectively.

References

Alvord ECJ, Loeser JD, Bailey WL, Copass MK (1972) Subarachnoid haemorrhage due to ruptured aneurysms. Archi Neurol 27: 273–284
Ask-Upmark E, Ingvar D (1950) A follow-up examination of 138 cases of subarachnoid haemorrhage. Acta Med Scand 138: 15–31
Awad IA (1996) Dural arteriovenous malformations. In: Carter LP, Spetzler RF (eds) Neurovasc Surg. McGraw-Hill, New York, pp 905–932
Awad IA, Little JR, Akarawi WP, Ahl J (1990) Intracranial dural arteriovenous malformations: factors predisposing to an aggressive neurological course. Neurosurg 72: 839–850

Bailes JE, Deeb ZL, Wilson JA et al. (1992) Inraoperative angiography and temporary balloon occlusion of the basilar artery as an adjunct to surgical clipping: technical note. Neurosurgery 30: 949–953

Borden JA, Wu JK, Shucart WA (1995) A proposed classification for spinal and cranial dural arteriovenous fistulous malformations and implications for treatment [published erratum appears in J Neurosurg 1995 82(4): 705–6]. Neurosurg 82: 166–179

Brown RD Jr, Wiebers DO, Forbes GS et al. (1988) The natural history of unruptured arteriovenous malformations. Neurosurg 68: 352–357

Celli P, Ferrante L, Palma L (1984). Cerebral arteriovenous malformations. Clinical features and outcome of treatment in children and in adults. Surgi Neurol 22: 43–49

Crawford PM, West CR, Chadwick DW, Shaw MDM (1986). Arteriovenous malformations of the brain: natural history in unoperated patients. J Neurol, Neurosurg & Psychiatr 49: 1–10

Crowell RM, Moayeri N, Ogilvy CS et al. (1995). Incidental aneurysms. In: Carter LP, Spetzler RF (eds) Neurovascular surgery. McGraw-Hill, New York pp 851–874

Davies MA, terBrugge K, Willinsky R, Coyne TJ, Saleh J, Wallace MC (1996). The validity of classification for the clinical presentation of intracranial dural arteriovenous fistulas. J Neurosurg 85: 830–837

Davies MA, Saleh J, terBrugge K, Wallace MC (1997a). The natural history and management of intracranial dural arteriovenous fistulae. Part 1: Benign lesions. Intervent Neuroradiol 3: 295–302

Davies MA, terBrugge K, Willinsky RA, Wallace MC (1997b). The natural history and management of intracranial dural arteriovenous fistulae Part 2: Aggressive lesions. Intervent Neuroradiol 3: 303–311

Dell S (1982) Asymptomatic cerebral aneurysm: assessment of its risk of rupture. Neurosurgery 10: 162–166

Dott NM (1969) Intracranial aneurysm formations. Clin Neurosurg 16: 1–15

Fleischer AS, Paton JM, Tindall GT (1975) Cerebral aneurysms of traumatic origin. Surg Neurol 4: 233–239

Forster DM, Steiner L, Hakanson S (1972) Arteriovenous malformations of the brain. J Neurosurg 37: 562–570

Fults D, Kelly DJL (1984) Natural history of arteriovenous malformations of the brain: a clinical study. Neurosurgery 15: 658–662

Gallagher JP (1964). Pilojection for intracranial aneurysms. Report of progress. J Neurosurg 21: 129–134

Garretson HD (1985) Intracranial arteriovenous malformations. In: Wilkins RH, Rengachary SA (eds) Neurosurgery. McGraw-Hill, New York, pp 1448–1458

Gerosa MA, Cappelloto P, Licata C (1981) Cerebral arteriovenous malformations in children (56 cases). Childs Brain 8: 356–371

Giombini S, Morello G (1978) Cavernous angiomas of the brain: Account of 14 personal cases and review of the literature. Acta Neurochirurgica (Wien) 40: 61–82

Girvin JP, Fox AJ, Vinuela F, Drake CG (1983). Intraoperative embolization of cerebral arteriovenous malformations in the awake patient. Clin Neurosurg 31: 188–247

Goldstein SJ, Tibbs PA (1981) Recurrent subarachnoid haemorrhage complicating cerebral arterial ectasia. J Neurosurg 55: 139–142

Graf CJ, Perret GE, Torresani T (1983) Bleeding from cerebral arteriovenous malformations as part of their natural history. J Neurosurg 58: 331–337

Guglielmi G, Vinuela F, Dion JE, Duckwiler G (1991) Electrothrombosis of saccular aneurysms via endovascular approach. Part 2: Preliminary clinical experience. J Neurosurg 75: 8–14

Hacein-Bey L, Cornolly ES, Mayer SA, Young WL, Pile-Spellman J, Solomon RA (1998) Complex intracranial aneurysms: Combined operative and endovascular approaches. Neurosurgery 43(6): 1304–1314

Heiskanen O (1970) Risk of rupture of a second aneurysms in a patient with multiple aneurysms. J Neurosurg 32: 295–299

Heiskanen O (1981) Risk of bleeding from unruptured aneurysm in cases with multiple intracranial aneurysms. J Neurosurg 55: 524–526

Heiskanen O (1986). Risk of surgery for unruptured aneurysms. J Neurosurg 65: 451–453

Heros RC, Korosue K, Diebold PM (1990) Surgical excision of cerebral arteriovenous malformations: late results. Neurosurgery 26: 570–577

Heros RC, Tu YK (1986). Unruptured arteriovenous malformations: a dilemma in surgical decision making. Clin Neurosurgery 33: 187–236

Higashida RT, Halbach VV, Barnwell SL et al. (1990) Treatment of intracranial aneurysms with preservation of the parent vessel: results of percutaneous balloon embolisation in 84 patients. Am J Neuroradiol 11: 633–640

Holtzman RNN, Brust JCM, Hughes JEO et al. (1995) Surgical management of infected intracranial aneurysms. In: Schmide KHN, Sweet WN (eds) Operative neurosurgical techniques. WB Saunders, London pp 1133–1153

Horton J, Chambers, W, Lyons S et al. (1990) Pregnancy and the risk of haemorrhage from cerebral arteriovenous malformations. Neurosurgery 27: 867–871

Joensen P (1984) Subarachnoid haemorrhage in an isolated population: Incidence on the Faroes during the period 1962-75. Stroke 15: 438-440

Kassel N, Torner JC (1983) Aneurysm rebleeding: a preliminary report from the co-operative aneurysm study. Neurosurgery 5: 479-481

Kassel N, Torner JC, Clarke Haley J et al. (1990). The international co-operative study on the timing of surgery. Part 1: Overall management results; Part 2: Surgical results. J Neurosurg 73: 18-47

Kelly DJL, Alexander E, Davis CJH, Maynard DC (1969) Intracranial arteriovenous malformations: clinical review and evaluation of brain scans. J Neurosurg 31: 422-428

Khayata MH, Wakhloo AK, Medkhour AM et al. (1995). Intravascular occlusion of cerebral arteriovenous malformations. In: Carter LP, Spetzler RF (eds) Neurovascular surgery. McGraw-Hill, New York, pp 957-978

Lasjaunias P, Chiu M, terBrugge K, Tolia A, Hurth M, Bernstein M (1986) Neurological manifestations of intracranial dural arterivenous malformations. J Neurosurg 64: 724-730

Luessenhop AJ (1985) Dural arteriovenous malformations. In: Wilkins RH, Rengachary SA (eds) Neurosurgery, McGraw-Hill, New York, pp 1473-1477

Malik GM, Pearce JM, Ausman JI, Mehta BA (1984) Dural arteriovenous malformations. Neurosurgery 15: 332-339

Manelfe C, Lasjaunias P, Halbach VV et al. (1990) Embolisation in the brain. In: Dandelinger RF, Rossi P, Kurdziel JC, Wallac S (eds) Interventional radiology. Thieme Medical Publishers, New York, pp 396-442

Martin, NA, Vinters, HV (1996) Arteriovenous malformations. In: Carter LP, Spetzler RF (eds) Neurovascular surgery. McGraw-Hill, New York, pp 875-903

Martin NA, Wilson CB (1984) Preoperative and postoperative care. Wilson CB, Stein BM (eds). Intracranial vascular malformations. Williams & Wilkins, Baltimore, pp 121-129

McCormick WF (1984). Pathology of vascular malformations of the brain. In: Wilson CB, Stein BM (eds) Intracranial vascular malformations. Williams & Wilkins, Baltimore, pp 44-63

McKissock W, Richardson AE, Walsh L (1965) Anterior commnicating artery aneurysms: a trail of conservative and surgical treatment. Lancet 1: 873-876

Menedelow AD, Erfurth A, Grossart K, Macpherson P (1987). Do cerebral arterioveneous malformations increase in size? J Neurol, Neurosurg Psychiatr 50: 980-987

Mizoi K, Takahashi A, Yoshimoto T, et al. (1993) Combined endovascular and neurosurgical approach for paraclinoid internal carotid artery aneurysms. Neurosurgery 33: 986-992

Mizoi K, Yoshimoto T, Takahashi A, Ogawa A (1994) Direct clipping of basilar trunk aneurysm using temporarily balloon occlusion. Neurosurgery 80: 230-236

Morcos JJ, Heros RC (1995) Supratentorial arteriovenous malformations. In: Carter LP, Spetzler RF (eds). Neurovascular surgery. McGraw-Hill, New York, pp 979-1004

Mori K, Murata T, Hashimoto N (1980) Clinical analysis of arteriovenous malformations in children. Childs Brain 6: 13-25

Moyes PD (1971) Surgical treatment of multiple aneurysms. J Neurosurg 35: 291-295

Mullan S, Raimondi AJ, Dobson G et al. (1965) Electrically induced thrombosis in intracranial aneurysms. J Neurosurg 22: 539-547

Nishioka H, Torner JC, Graf CJ et al. (1984) Co-operative study of intracranial aneurysms and subarachnoid haemorrhage: a long term prognostic study. II. Ruptured intracranial aneurysms managed conservatively. Archi Neurol 41: 1142-1146

Numaguchi Y, Kitamura K, Fukui M et al. (1982) Intracranial venous angiomas. Surg Neurol 18: 193-202

Ohman J, Heiskanen O (1989) Timing of operation for ruptured supratentorial aneurysms: a prospective randomised study. J Neurosurg 70: 55-60

Ojemann RG (1985) Infectious intracranial aneurysms. In: Flein JM, Flamm ES (eds) Cerebrovascular disease. Springer-Verlag, New York, pp 1047-1060

Ondra SL, Troupp H, George ED, Schwab K (1990) The natural history of symptomatic arteriovenous malformations of the brain. J Neurosurg 73: 387-391

Pakarinen S (1967) Incidence, aetiology, and prognosis of primary subarachnoid haemorrhage. A study based on 589 cases diagnosed in a defined urban population during a defined period. Acta Neurol Scand 43: Suppl-28

Perret G, Nishioka H (1966) Arteriovenous malfornations: an analysis of 545 cases of cranio-cerebral malformations and fistulae reported to the cooperative study. J Neurosurg 25: 467-490

Porter PJ, Willinsky RA, Harper W, Wallace MC (1997) Cerebral cavernous malformations: natural history and prognosis after clinical deterioration with or without haemorrhage. J Neurosurg 87: 190-197

Redekop G, Ferguson G (1995). Intracranial aneurysms. In: Carter LP, Spetzler R (eds) Neurovascular surgery. McGraw-Hill, New York, pp 625-648

Robinson JL, Hall CS, Sedzmir CB (1974) Arteriovenous malformations, aneurysms and pregnancy. J Neurosurg 41: 63-70

Rosenorn J, Eskesen V, Schmidt K et al. (1987) Clinical features and outcome in 1076 patients with ruptured intracranial saccular aneurysms: prospective constructive study. Br J Neurosurg 1: 33-46

Rothfus WE, Albright AL, Cassey KF et al. (1984) Cerebellar venous angioma: "Benign" entity? Am J Neuroradiol 6: 61-66

Sahs AL, Perret GE, Locksley HB et al. (1969) Intracranial aneurysms and subarachnoid haemorrhage: co-operative study. Lippincott, Philadelphia.

Samson DS, Batjer HH (1991) Preoperative evaluation of the risk/benefit ratio for arteriovenous malformations of the brain. In: Wilkins RH, Rengachary SS (eds) Neurosurgery update II. Vascular, spinal paediatric and functional neurosurgery. McGraw-Hill, New York, pp 129-133

Sarwar M, McCormick WF (1978) Intracerebral venous angioma: Case report and review. Arch Neurol 35: 323-325

Saveland H, Hillman J, Brandt L et al. (1992) A prospective study from neurosurgical units in Sweden during a 1-year period. J of Neurosurg 76: 729-734

Scott N, Ballantine HT Jr (1972) Spontaneous thrombosis in a giant middle cerebral aneurysms. J Neurosurg 37: 361-363

Sedzmir CB, Robinson J (1973) Intracranial haemorrhage in children and adolescents. J Neurosurg 38: 269-281

Senegor M, Dohrmann GJ, Wolmann RL (1983) Venous angiomas of the posterior fossa should be considered as anomalous venous drainage. Surgi Neurol 19: 26-32

Sparrow OC (1998) Cavernous malformations. Br J Neurosurg 12(6): 517-520

Sonntag VK, Yuan RH, Stein BM (1977) Giant intracranial aneurysms: a review of 13 cases. Surgi Neurol 8: 81-84

Torner JC (1985) Natural history of intracranial vascular malformations: A review. Neurosurgery 16: 421.

Voigt K, Yasargil MG (1976) Cerebral cavernous haemangiomas or cevernomas. Incidence, pathology, localisation, diagnosis, clinical features and treatment. Review of the literature and report of an unusual case. Neurochirurgia 19: 59-68

Wascher TM, Spetzler RF (1995) Cavernous malformations of the brainstem. In: Carter LP, Spetzler RF (eds) Neurovascular surgery. McGraw-Hill, New York, pp 541-555

Weinand ME (1996) Arteriovenous malformations and epilepsy. Neurovascular surgery. McGraw-Hill, New York, pp 933-956

Weir B. Aneurysms affecting the nervous system (1987). Williams & Wilkins, Baltimore.

Wiebers DO (1998) Unruptued intracranial aneurysms – risk of rupture and risks of surgical intervention. New Engl J Med 339: 1725-1733

Wiebers DO, Whisnant JP, Sundt TM Jr, O'Fallon WM (1987) The significance of unruptured intracranial saccular aneurysms. J Neurosurg 66: 23-29

Wilkins RH (1985) Natural history of intracranial vascular malformations: a review. Neurosurgery 16: 421-430

Winn HR, Almaani WS, Berga SL, Richardson AE (1983) The long term outcome in patients with multiple aneurysms: incidence of late haemorrhage and implications for treatment of incidental aneurysms. J Neurosurgery 59: 642-651

Wirth FP (1986) Surgical treatment of intracranial aneurysms. Clini Neurosurg 33: 125-135

Wirth FP, Laws ER Jr, Piepgras DG, Scott RM (1983) Surgical treatment of intracranial aneurysms. Neurosurgery 12: 507-511

Chapter 2

Interventional Neuroradiology: Techniques in Embolisation of Cerebral Aneurysms and Arteriovenous Malformations

Anil R. Gholkar and Joti J. Bhattacharya

Introduction

Modern techniques in interventional neuroradiology for treating vascular lesions have followed developments in catheter and guidewire technology, and are still evolving. The combination of modern microcatheters and digital angiography equipment, with a better understanding of cerebral haemodynamics has made a wide variety of lesions accessible to treatment.

Although focusing on technique in this chapter, the clinical nature of interventional neuroradiology bears repeated stressing. The selection of patients for endovascular treatment of aneurysm or arteriovenous malformation (AVM) requires the experience and judgement of neuroradiologist and neurosurgeon, and the success of the treatment requires a dedicated team including radiographers, nurses, anaesthetists and intensive care unit staff, in addition to the neuroradiologist.

Poor risk patients and inaccessible aneurysms have been the impetus for the development of alternatives to surgical clipping. Surgery, however remains the standard against which other treatments must be compared. Giant aneurysms have long been treated by ligation of the parent vessel and early endovascular treatments achieved the same result using detachable balloons (Serbinenko, 1974). Early attempts at surgical intrasaccular treatment of aneurysms in the 1960s included the technique of pilojection: the transmural placement of sterile hog or horse hairs into the sac, to induce thrombosis, using a pneumatic gun at open craniotomy (Gallagher, 1964). Placement of metal electrodes or wire within the aneurysm by open or stereotactic methods, for electrothrombosis (Mullan, 1974; Hosobuchi, 1979) or iron filings held in place by a magnetic probe (Alksne & Fingerhut, 1965) were also tried. Luessenhop and Velazquez (1964) reported the first attempted endovascular catheterisation of an aneurysm sac. The first successful endovascular obliteration of an intracranial aneurysm with preservation of the parent artery was described by Serbinenko (1974) in the former Soviet Union, using a detachable latex balloon. In the 1980s other workers used silastic or silicone balloons sometimes filled with methacrylate glue (Goto et al., 1988). Mechanically detached platinum microcoils were first reported by Hilal (1988). The current explosion of interest in endovascular treatment of aneurysms followed Guglielmi's introduction of the electrolytically detachable microcoil in 1991 (Guglielmi et al., 1991 a, b).

Endovascular treatment of cerebral arteriovenous malformations was undertaken by Luessenhop and colleagues (1960). Plastic microspheres were injected following exposure of the cervical internal carotid artery, relying on blood flow to carry them to the site of the lesion. Subsequent methods have employed polyvinylacetate (PVA) particles, silk, detachable balloons and coils. A great advancement has been the introduction of cyanoacrylate glue (in particular the newer N-butyl-2-cyanoacrylate (NBCA)) which can permeate into the nidus of the AVM and completely occlude it (Putman & Chaloupka, 1996). Endovascular techniques have also contributed greatly to the understanding of the haemodynamic properties of AVMs.

Equipment

Angiography Unit

Angiographic equipment of high quality and good reliability is mandatory for the safe and successful performance of these procedures. The main requirements are for digital subtraction angiography, fine resolution, high frame rates (many units allow 6 or more frames per second) and a roadmapping facility. In addition equipment should not be so bulky as to preclude ready access to the patient in an emergency. Most centres currently use C-arm equipment; the apparatus may have a rotational angiography facility in which the C-arm pivots around the patient during a single contrast injection, simulating a three-dimensional effect. A real-time three-dimensional effect is available on some units. Biplanar digital fluoroscopy while much more expensive and reducing access to the patient is useful and shortens procedure duration.

Magnetic resonance angiography (MRA) and computed tomography angiography (CTA) are now routinely available. Improvment in resolution of these techniques has made it possible to asses the neck of complex aneurysms in three dimensions.

Guiding Catheters

Guiding catheters are available from most major manufacturers (Putman & Chaloupka, 1996). The ideal guiding catheter should be long enough to allow distal positioning, for example in the internal carotid artery just below the skull base allowing more secure subsequent microcatheterisation. It should give good torque control and may have an angled tip avoiding the need for catheter exchanges. The distal portion should be supple and atraumatic and the catheter should have a large lumen permitting good roadmaps while the microcatheter is in situ. The sizes most commonly used range from 5 F to 7 F (Figure 2.1). Great care must clearly be taken in using these large calibre, relatively stiff and potentially traumatic catheters.

Microcatheters

Microcatheters are of two main types: steerable and flow-guided, and are usually passed through guiding catheters of 5F to 7F. Steerable microcatheters are designed to track over guidewires. They taper over their length from a stiffer proximal section conferring torquability and pushability to a progressively more supple distal portion,

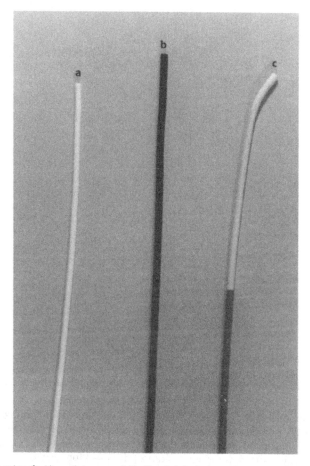

Fig. 2.1. A wide variety of guiding catheters are available. These include simple straight catheters such as the widely used 5F Balt **a**, which we favour for AVMs, and shapeable catheters such as the Fasguide 6F and 7F which have soft atraumatic tips **b**. Large calibre angled-tip 6F Envoy catheters **c**, are particularly useful for aneurysm cases. Their large internal lumen, even when partially occupied by a microcatheter, allows sufficient space for effective road-map injections, although their relative stiffness demands great care in use.

the tip of which can be steamed into a curve if desired. Several manufacturers produce microcatheters usually designed for use with their own wires and embolic devices. We use mainly the Tracker range of microcatheters (Target Therapeutics, Fremont, CA). The Tracker 18 has an inner diameter of 0.45 mm, and naturally must be used with smaller guidewires (such as 0.4 or 0.35 mm), its stiffer proximal portion is 3F and tapers to a distal 2. 5F (Kikuchi et al., 1987). Versions are available with one or two metallic tip-markers, the two tip-marker catheter being used with detachable microcoils (Figure 2.2). A newer generation of catheters (Tracker 18 MX) have shafts of braided construction which are less likely to kink in tortuous vessels. Further refinements include hydrophilic coatings (Fas-Tracker) intended to reduce friction also in tortuous vessels and a larger lumen model (HiFlow). A smaller calibre Tracker 10 catheter with an internal diameter of 0.25 mm is also available. These

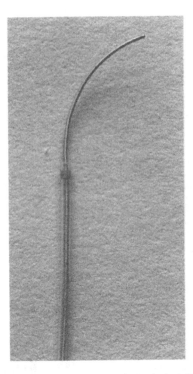

Fig. 2.2. The distal portion of a Tracker 18 microcatheter with a guidewire, the tip of which bears a shaped curve, projecting beyond it. Note the single metallic tip marker on this catheter. Catheters for use with GDCs bear two tip markers.

steerable catheters may be used with many embolic agents including detachable microcoils, PVA particles, cyanoacrylate liquid adhesive and premounted detachable balloons. A similar two tip-marker catheter tapering from 3F to 2F is available from Balt (MAG 3F/2F, Balt, Montmorency, France) designed for use with Balt MDS coils. A number of other manufacturers now produce microcatheters. Prowler (Cordis Endovascular Systems), Jetstream (Medtronic Micro Interventional Systems, MIS) and Turbo Tracker (Target Therapeutics) microcatheters have improved our ability for distal catheterisation of tortuous vessels, while maintaining internal lumen and reducing friction. Care should, however, be taken while using these microcatheters as there is risk of perforation of vessels or aneurysms. Steerable catheters are suitable for a wide range of lesions and locations. For the more distal, smaller, tortuous vessels often encountered in cerebral AVMs, however, loss of torque control and increased friction may make attempts at catheterisation less safe.

Flow-guided microcatheters are useful for distal catheterisation of previously inaccessible AVMs. In contrast to steerable catheters, they are carried distally by blood flow, tending to follow the course of greatest flow, usually into the feeding vessels of the AVM. Not requiring guidewires, they are less traumatic. Flow-guided catheters are also tapered with a long floppy distal portion (Dion et al., 1989). We use the Magic series (Balt) which have proximal 3F shafts with distal silastic 1.8F or 1.5F sections (Figure 2.3). These are available with standard tips and olive tips, the latter consisting of a slightly bulbous weighted tip intended to reach more distal branches. These catheters will also accept a steamed curve and injecting pulses of

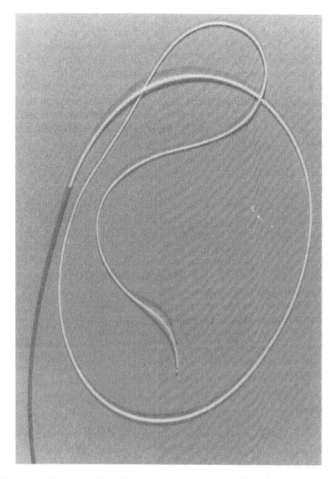

Fig. 2.3. A flow-directed Magic microcatheter. Note the composite construction and the extreme flexibility of the distal silastic portion.

contrast medium through them has the effect of deflecting the catheter tip slightly. This will free the catheter, if it becomes impacted on the vessel side-wall, allowing it to resume its flow directed course. Deflecting the tip in this way may also allow the catheter to enter a desired vessel at a branch point. These catheters allow no torque control and have minimal pushability. A hydrophilic coated guidewire may be inserted into the proximal stiff portion of the catheter, not to allow steering but rather to allow some proximal pushing. Some users attempt to reduce friction between catheter and vessel wall further by applying a silicone spray, wiped over the outer surface of the shaft. Magic catheters are only used with liquid adhesive.

Introduction of ultralite (Medtronic Micro Interventional Systems, MIS) and spinnaker (Target Therapeutics) flow-guided hydrophilic microcatheters have significantly improved our ability to catheterise the AVM nidus. Both of these catheters will take hydrophilic 010 guide wires allowing distal placement of microcatheter. We now frequently start with one of the above two catheters when treating an AVM.

Other flow-directed catheters are available, some with hydrophilic coating. These include Sense microcatheters (Nycomed, Paris, France) tapering from 2.8F to1.9F, and Eddy infusion catheters (Boston Scientific Corporation, Scimed, Maple Grove, MN) tapering from either 2.7F to 2.2F, or 2.4F to 2.2F. The larger size Eddy catheter may be used with a steerable guidewire up to 0.4 mm, while the Sense catheter is designed for flow-guidance, or use with a 0.3 mm guidewire. All of these highly supple, flow-guided catheters are easily damaged by guidewires and the decision to use a wire must, therefore, be carefully considered. Smaller calibre flow-guided catheters are for use with liquid agents, while larger catheters can be used with a variety of embolic materials.

Guidewires

Most guidewires for microcatheters have a stainless steel monofilament shaft tipped with a highly flexible, shapeable platinum coil. They are available from several manufacturers to complement their own brand of microcatheters. We use mainly the Dasher series (Target Therapeutics): the Dasher 14 and Dasher 10 use core wires of 0.35 and 0.251 mm, respectively. Core wires of 0.41 mm are also available. All of these wires taper progressively with either a step-grind or transitionless grind profile, aiding steerability and pushability proximally but maintaining distal flexibility. Many wires have Teflon or hydrophilic coatings and newer developments include the use of highly elastic nitinol core wire in an attempt to reduce kinking and improve flexibility. In spite of their shapeable tips, all of these wires tend to lose any added curve with time in the body, because of the relatively poor memory of the distal coil. Torque devices may be attached to the distal portion of the wire to aid steering further.

Embolic Agents

This section is concerned principally with detachable microcoils for aneurysm treatment and liquid adhesives for AVM embolisation. Other embolic agents and detachable balloons are considered briefly.

Detachable microcoils have superceded balloons in the endosaccular treatment of cerebral aneurysms and are available from several manufacturers. The Guglielmi detachable coil (GDC, Target Therapeutics) is the most widely used system at present and was reported by Guglielmi et al. (1991a, b). It gained approval for general use in Europe and subsequently in the USA in 1995. The platinum coil is soldered to the end of a stainless steel pusher wire and detached by electrolysis using a 1 mA DC proprietary power supply. The GDCs are constructed from a fine platinum stock wire, from 0.05 to 0.1 mm diameter wound into a primary helix of 0.38 mm for GDC 18 or 0.25 mm for GDC 10 coils. The wire is then wound into a secondary helix of diameter ranging from 2 to 20 mm (10mm with GDC 10), and length ranging from 4 cm (2cm with GDC 10) to 30 cm for use in aneurysms of varying size). The shape of the secondary helix is stored in the circular memory of the coil allowing it to reform as it emerges from the microcatheter. Coil technology is continuously evolving: soft coils are now available, constructed from a finer platinum stock wire they exert less radial force and may be preferred for use in acutely ruptured aneurysms. The diameter of the first turn is smaller (75%) than that of the rest of the coil in the new 2 D coils (Target Therapeutics) which may reduce endosaccular trauma and also prevent the leading end of the coil from emerging into the parent vessel. More complex three-dimensional shapes, and coated coils with increased thrombogenicity are being developed.

Several types of mechanically detachable coil are also produced (Moret et al., 1993; Marks et al., 1994). These include mechanical detachable system (MDS, Balt) coils, made from tungsten, and featuring ball and socket attachment to a pusher wire. They have the advantage of being cheaper than GDCs, especially valuable with large aneurysms, and being made of tungsten are of inherently higher thrombogenicity than the platinum coils. Conversely the detachment mechanism is less sure and can be difficult to achieve in vivo, the coils are stiffer, exerting potentially more force on the inner walls of the aneurysm during placement, and there is much greater friction between the coil and the inner wall of the catheter. In addition MDS coils must be manually preloaded onto the pusher wire before use, a rather laborious procedure. Premounted coils are available but are more expensive.

Currently NBCA monomer is the most widely used polymerising agent for AVM embolisation that appears to result in permanent occlusion (Wikholm, 1995). This is marketed under the name Histoacryl blue (B. Braun, Melsungen, Germany) supplied in 1-ml ampoules, and was designed originally as a tissue adhesive. Injected in liquid form, it can penetrate into the nidus of an AVM, polymerisation occurring within seconds on contact with ionic solutions. Prior to injection, NBCA is usually mixed with the oily contrast medium iophendylate (Lipiodol). This renders the NBCA radio-opaque and also slows its polymerisation time, which lengthens as the proportion of Lipiodol increases. Further opacification may be obtained by the addition of tungsten or tantalum powder. Goggles should be worn during preparation of the NBCA mixture to reduce the chance of splash injury to the eyes. Before embolising, the microcatheter must be carefully flushed with 5% dextrose solution to prevent polymerisation within the catheter.

Other embolic agents have been used in the treatment of AVMs. These include PVA particles, silk suture, concentrated ethanol and ethylene vinyl alcohol copolymer (EVAL). For a full discussion of these and other agents the reader is referred to other specialist texts (Dion, 1992). Detachable balloons (Figure 2.4) are currently used mainly for parent vessel occlusion, in the presence of otherwise untreatable aneurysms and are produced by several manufacturers (ITC, San Francisco, CA; Balt, Montmorency, France; Ingenor, Paris, France). Both silicone and latex balloons are available and must be mounted manually on the tip of a microcatheter (such as a Tracker 18). Balloons are inflated with contrast medium and detached usually by gentle traction on the microcatheter. They have self sealing valves that close as the catheter is withdrawn, leaving the balloon inflated. Silicone is semipermeable and care must, therefore, be taken to use only isotonic contrast medium for inflation. These manufacturers also produce non-detachable balloon catheters which are safer for temporary occlusion.

General Principles and Vascular Access

The selection of patients for endovascular treatment of aneurysm or AVM requires the experience and judgement of neuroradiologist and neurosurgeon and the success of the treatment requires a dedicated team including radiographers, nurses, anaesthetists and intensive care unit staff in addition to the neuroradiologist. It is important for the interventional neuroradiologist to obtain informed consent for all procedures. This of course includes a discussion of the natural history of the disease

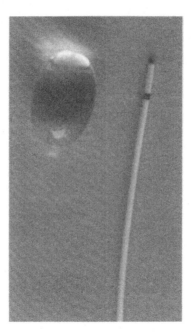

Fig. 2.4. An inflated micro-balloon alongside its dedicated delivery catheter. The catheter tip is inserted into the projecting flutter valve on the balloon. As the catheter is withdrawn from the inflated balloon the valve closes.

and the alternative treatments available. The procedure itself should be outlined and in the case of microcoil embolisation of cerebral aneurysms, the newness of the treatment and consequent uncertainty regarding long-term results must be explained. Complications, including risk of stroke and death, must also be addressed and their acceptance detailed in the patient's records.

Additional medical therapy may be prescribed on admission. This may include calcium channel blocking drugs such as nimodipine, in an attempt to reduce the likelihood of vasospasm, corticosteroids such as dexamethasone, to reduce cerebral swelling, and H_2 receptor antagonists such as ranitidine to reduce gastrointestinal side effects of steroid therapy. Preoperative investigations should include full blood count and coagulation studies. Access to intensive care or high dependency unit beds for postoperative care is ideal but not always available.

The common femoral artery is the preferred site for cannulation for aneurysm and AVM embolisation. The patient's groin is shaved, prepped and draped in the normal manner for angiography. Following local anaesthetic infiltration (a long-acting agent is preferable because of the length of some procedures), a small scalpel incision is made over the common femoral artery and the latter is then punctured using the Seldinger technique. A large introducer sheath, usually 6F or 7F is inserted into the artery over the guidewire and sutured to the skin. The sheath sidearm is continually flushed with heparinised saline from a pressure bag.

A guiding catheter is then advanced distally into the desired vessel under fluoroscopic guidance, an optimal position being confirmed by test injection of contrast medium. A preprimed rotating haemostatic valve, with all air bubbles carefully expelled, and sidearm connected to a second pressure bag containing heparinised saline, is now attached to the hub of the catheter. The guiding catheter is now also continuously flushed. A three-way tap attached to the sidearm of the rotating haemostatic valve permits contrast medium injection through the guiding catheter which is now ready for introduction of a microcatheter.

Endovascular Treatment of Cerebral Aneurysms

Several therapeutic options currently exist for the treatment of intracranial aneurysms. The particular treatment selected depends on a number of factors: principally the clinical situation of the patient (subarachnoid haemorrhage or unruptured aneurysm), the nature of the aneurysm (including size, shape and location) and the expertise available. Management options include: conservative treatment, surgical clipping or wrapping , surgical ligation or endovascular occlusion of parent vessel, with or without internal carotid to external carotid bypass, and endovascular intrasaccular occlusion of the aneurysm.

Parent Vessel Occlusion

Giant cavernous carotid and vertebrobasilar aneurysms present special problems for both neurosurgeon and interventional neuroradiologist. Direct surgical treatment may be difficult or impossible while endovascular coiling of giant aneurysms may also be impossible because of a wide necked or fusiform lesion, or commonly show a suboptimal outcome because of coil compaction and recannulation. Giant aneurysms also require a large number of coils for complete occlusion, which may cause resource problems. Hunterian ligation of the internal or common carotid artery has long been the preferred surgical treatment for giant cavernous aneurysms.

Endovascular balloon occlusion of the parent artery proximal to the aneurysm offers the same protection from haemorrhage (Figure 2.5) but has several advantages

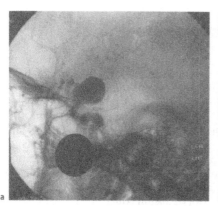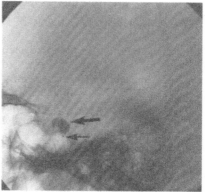

Fig. 2.5. A giant, partially thrombosed intracranial aneurysm was demonstrated on CT in this elderly patient with visual symptoms. Balloon occlusion of the left ICA was performed. The angiogram demonstrates filling of the residual lumen of the aneurysm. Note the much larger calcified rim in part **a**. A detachable balloon has been maneouvred into the cavernous segment of the ICA and inflated with isotonic contrast medium (large arrow) completely occluding the vessel. The balloon has not yet been detached and the microcatheter with its tip marker are visible (small arrows) in **b**. A second balloon was subsequently placed in the petrous portion of the ICA.

(Hodes et al., 1991). The procedure is performed by the usual transfemoral approach under local anaesthesia, allowing continuous monitoring of an awake patient. The patient's ability to tolerate occlusion of the parent vessel must be assessed before definitive treatment and a balloon test occlusion can be performed at the same sitting. A large calibre (7F) guiding catheter is introduced into the desired vessel and the balloon catheter, bearing the premounted silicone balloon, is advanced through this and positioned fluoroscopically. At this stage the patient is fully heparinised. The test occlusion is performed by inflating the balloon with contrast medium proximal to the aneurysm. The patients neurological status is carefully monitored over the next 20 to 30 minutes, the balloon being immediately deflated if the patient develops a neurological deficit. Some authors recommend provoked hypotension to two thirds of the mean arterial pressure for 20 minutes during the test period; electroencephalograph (EEG) monitoring or assessment of cerebral perfusion by single position emission CT (SPECT) or xenon CT may also be performed.

If the patient tolerates the test occlusion, the balloon is detached, usually close to the aneurysm to prevent a long column of thrombus forming, for example in the petrous portion of the internal carotid astery (ICA) for a cavernous or internal carotid bifurcation aneurysm. A second safety balloon is usually placed below the first. Our policy is to heparinise fully all these patients for 48 hours after the occlusion.

Peroperative Temporary Balloon Occlusion of Parent Vessel

Temporary vessel occlusion is sometimes necessary to achieve proximal control, with surgically difficult aneurysms such as those of the basilar or ophthalmic arteries. A non-detachable balloon catheter may be placed in the appropriate vessel immediately prior to surgery, if the parent vessel is not accessible for a temporary clip (Aspoas et al., 1993). The balloon can then be inflated as required during the operation.

Endosaccular Occlusion of Aneurysms

Coil occlusion is now the preferred endovascular treatment for cerebral aneurysms. Current microcoils have the great advantage over previous systems of being attached to pusher wires which allow withdrawal of the coil if optimal placement cannot be achieved. Detachment from the pusher wire may be electrolytic as in the widely used Guglielmi detachable coil (GDC, Target Therapeutics, Fremont, CA), or mechanical as in the Mechanical Detachable Coil (MDS, Balt, France) and Interlocking Detachable Coil (IDC, Target Therapeutics) Detachable balloons are no longer favoured in most centres because of higher risks of distal migration, recanalisation and rupture. The success of Russian workers with balloon occlusion has not been generally reproducible. The platinum Guglielmi detachable coil (GDC, Target), is the most widely used system for coil occlusion (Guglielmi et al., 1991a, b).

Patient Selection

Selection of patients for GDC embolisation demands close co-operation between neurosurgeon and interventionist and will usually follow diagnostic angiography.

The suitability of the lesion in terms of its size, location and neck are assessed. The angiogram should give a good view of the neck of the aneurysm in profile, projected clear of the parent vessel, which is often difficult in the case of middle cerebral artery trifurcation lesions. Giant aneurysms (larger than 25 mm diameter) frequently show recannulation following coil embolisation, with compaction of coils into the mural thrombus. We no longer favour endosaccular treatment for these lesions. Ironically, early experience has shown that aneurysms which are the best candidates for open surgery; small lesions with narrow necks are also the best candidates for embolisation. Endovascular treatment may be deemed preferable because the patient is otherwise unfit for surgery or because the lesion may be in a surgically inaccessible location, eg posterior fossa or infraclinoid ICA. The state of the aneurysm: ruptured or unruptured and patient preference may also have a bearing. Prospective randomised trials are currently being performed comparing GDC embolisation with surgical clipping.

Preparation

Informed consent for the procedure is obtained as described above. Standard medical treatment for subarachnoid haemorrhage is continued if appropriate. Close co-operation with the attending anaesthetist is necessary throughout. Embolisation is commonly performed under general anaesthesia to minimise movement; however cooperative patients may only require light sedation. The patients pulse, blood pressure, electrocardiogram and oxygen saturation are constantly monitored; we also always insert a urinary catheter. A full range of sizes of microcoils in addition to delivery catheters, is obviously a prerequisite.

Technique

Vascular access is obtained and a suitable guiding catheter positioned in the appropriate vessel as described above. Measurements of the aneurysm fundus (and neck if necessary) diameters are conveniently made at this stage (see below). The selection of the microcatheter/guidewire combination depends on several factors including vessel tortuosity, the size and appearance of the parent vessel from which the aneurysm arises, the size of the aneurysm itself and on the type of microcoil required. Curves are placed on the guidewire, and also on the microcatheter by steam heating. After flushing with heparinised saline, the microcatheter is preloaded with the guidewire. A second preprimed rotating haemostatic valve, with its sidearm connected to a third pressure bag containing heparinised saline, is attached to the hub of the microcatheter. The preloaded guidewire projects back through the valve. Continuous flushing of the microcatheter is started and the whole assembly is introduced through the haemostatic valve on the guiding catheter. The femoral sheath, guiding catheter and microcatheter are thus all continuously flushed with heparinised saline throughout the procedure. Vigilance must be maintained throughout the procedure to prevent, or remove, blood refluxing into the haemostatic valves. At this stage systemic anticoagulation of the patient is commenced. It is important to monitor the state of anticoagulation of the patient during the procedure, giving further doses of heparin as required.

The guidewire and microcatheter are now advanced beyond the guiding catheter under fluoroscopic control. The digital "road map" facility is useful in guiding the microcatheter carefully into the aneurysm (Figure 2.6). The tip of the microcatheter

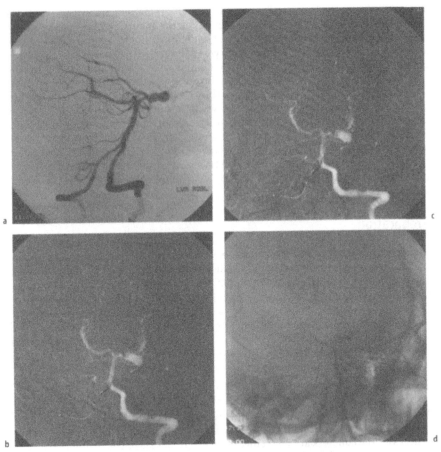

Fig. 2.6. Angiograms showing guide + microcath and roadmap. **a** Digital roadmap allows the aneurysm to be approached safely by guidewire and microcatheter. **b** Position of guidewire and microcatheter clearly demonstrated on the roadmap. **c** Microcatheter positioned within aneurysm sac. **d** First turn of the coil deployed. **e** First coil detached. **f** Last coil being delivered into aneurysm. **g** Post embolisation image showing complete occlusion of aneurysm.

is positioned within the aneurysm sac taking care not to allow the guidewire to project beyond the catheter where it could pierce the aneurysm wall. Test injections of contrast via the guiding catheter may be performed as necessary to confirm a satisfactory position. Injections through the microcatheter while its tip lies within the aneurysm are not recommended because of the risk of rupture, or dislodgement of thrombus.

Selection of the appropriate coil depends on the size and appearance of the aneurysm. The diameter of the lesion can be assessed by cursor measurements calibrated to the diameter of the guiding catheter, a method available on most modern angiography units. Alternatively calibration can be from markers taped to the skin surface allowing for magnification effects. Knowledge of the usual diameter of the parent vessel allows an estimate of the aneurysm size also. For acutely ruptured aneurysms we use GDC-soft, while for small lesions we use GDC-10.

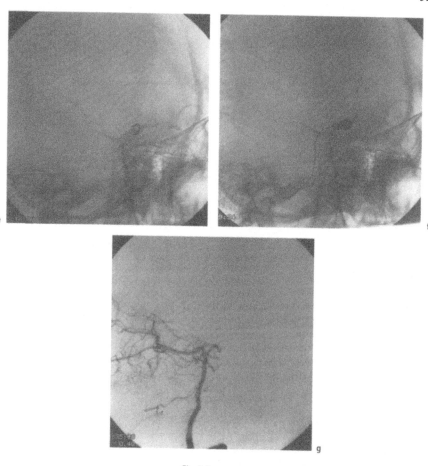

Fig. 2.6. e–g

Choosing the correct length of coil is largely a matter of experience. Longer and larger diameter coils are placed first with progressive reduction in size and length as packing proceeds.

The chosen coil is then advanced into the aneurysm under fluoroscopy, with road mapping if necessary. When the coil is satisfactorily positioned, as determined by fluoroscopy and further contrast runs, the decision is taken to detach it. This may be achieved electrolytically with GDC, or mechanically with MDS or IDC. Further contrast runs allow determination of the degree of obliteration of the sac and whether further coils are needed.

When the final coil has been detached, the microcatheter is withdrawn carefully from the aneurysm and removed. A postembolisation angiogram is performed via the guiding catheter, which is then withdrawn (Figure 2.7). We do not favour routine heparinisation after embolisation and when coagulation has returned to normal, the femoral introducer sheath is removed. Systemic heparinisation may be continued if there is deemed to be a high risk of thromboembolism, for example if a loop of coil projects through a wide neck into the vessel lumen.

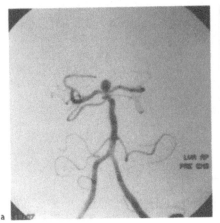 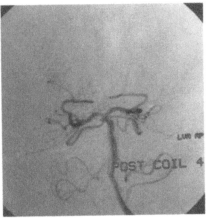

Fig. 2.7. Angiogram revealed a basilar bifurcation aneurysm in this 40-year-old woman who presented with subarachnoid haemorrhage **a**. A further tiny 1–2 mm aneurysm arises from the basilar /superior cerebellar artery junction. The basilar tip aneurysm was completely occluded with GDCs **b**. The other lesion is being kept under observation.

The patient is returned preferably to the high dependency or intensive care unit for close observation; the neuroradiologist should be closely involved in the postoperative care. The patient is kept hydrated and a normal blood pressure maintained in an uncomplicated case. Standard medical treatment for subarachnoid haemorrhage is continued if necessary. Following elective embolisation the patient is usually discharged after two or three days. A first check angiogram is usually arranged at 6 months after the embolisation.

Special Techniques for Wide-necked Aneurysms

Placement of coils in wide-necked aneurysms may be difficult and sometimes impossible. A technique using a non-detachable balloon at the neck of the aneurysm has been used by some interventionists for appropriate lesions (Moret et al., 1997). The balloon catheter is manoeuvred across the neck of the aneurysm. The microcatheter is placed in the sac of the aneurysm following which the balloon is inflated to block the wide neck. The coil is now delivered. Following this, the balloon is deflated to check the stability of the coil and identify any herniation into the parent vessel. If the coils position appears safe it is now detached. The procedure is repeated for further coils as necessary. Aneurysms may occasionally be encountered which are inaccessible to complete surgical clipping and yet are too wide-necked for safe coiling alone. Surgical clipping even if unable to completely occlude the aneurysm may narrow the neck sufficiently to allow coil embolisation (Marks et al., 1995).

Complications

Complications may arise during or after the procedure. As with any angiographic procedure, contrast medium reactions, haemorrhage, dissection, thromboembolism and infective complications may occur at the puncture site. More specific complications include perforation of vessels by the microguidewire. This is better avoided by careful scrutiny and manipulation during catheterisation, but, if recognised and the guidewire withdrawn, is usually uneventful. Rupture of the aneurysm during catheterisation or coiling is more serious, and fortunately rare. In this situation the desire to pull out the catheter should be resisted. Heparinisation should be reversed and if possible the coiling should be continued to occlude the perforation site. CT will usually be necessary to assess the size of the bleed and any resulting haematoma, hydrocephalus or raised intracranial pressure will require the appropriate neurosurgical treatment. Occlusion of the parent vessel may occur, for example if the coil prolapses into the vessel lumen. This may or may not be symptomatic. Prolapsed loops may sometimes be pushed back into the aneurysm by inflating a nondetachable balloon across its neck. Failure of normal detachment and premature withdrawal of the pusher wire, can result in stretching and unwinding of the coil, and a long length of platinum wire extending into the parent vessel. In this situation it is sometimes possible to snare the free end and position it in a less critical vessel such as the external carotid artery. Cerebral vasospasm may be treated with antispasmodic agents such as papaverine (Clouston et al., 1995) or by angioplasty (Eskridge et al., 1994), while distal thromboembolism may be treatable with thrombolytic agents. Postprocedural complications include rebleeding and vasospasm, which can be identified on repeat angiography or CT. Repeated embolic episodes may require long-term warfarin treatment.

Endovascular Treatment of Arteriovenous Malformations

Treatment options for cerebral arteriovenous malformations include surgery, stereotactic radiosurgery and embolisation either alone or in combination. The goal of treatment is usually complete obliteration of the lesion and requires multidisciplinary consultation. The choice of treatment depends on the size, location and microanatomical features, or angioarchitecture of the lesion, as defined by diagnostic angiography. Various grading systems have been devised in an attempt to rationalise treatment, the one proposed by Spetzler and Martin (1986) being widely used (Table 2.1), although this is more applicable to surgical than endovascular management.

Table 2.1. Spetzler and Martin grading for cerebral arteriovenous malformations. Grade from I to V (Roman numerals) = total number of points from three factors

Factor	Points
AVM size	
Small <3 cm	1
Medium 3–6 cm	2
Large >6 cm	3
Functional eloquence of lesion	
Non-eloquent	0
Eloquent	1
Venous drainage complex	
Surface cortical only	0
Deep or galenic	1

As in all areas of endovascular therapy, the exact place of the various treatment options is not well defined and continues to evolve. Small AVMs (grade I–II) in non-eloquent areas can safely be excised. Surgical morbidity becomes an important factor with high grade lesions, which may be inoperable, and embolisation and radiosurgery may be considered alone or in combination. Such grading systems notwithstanding, each lesion must clearly be assessed individually.

A variety of embolic agents have been used for treating AVMs, including PVA particles, coils and balloons. Currently the favoured agents are cyanoacrylate adhesives which polymerise on contact with ionic solutions (see previous discussion).

Patient Selection

Following initial CT or MRI, angiography reveals the morphology of the AVM. High-flow lesions will require faster frame rates than usual (from 3–6 frames per second). On the arterial side there may be ectasia, and aneurysms both on the feeding vessel and on the circle of Willis secondary to the increased flow. The nidus, or core of the AVM, consisting of numerous, thin-walled, tortuous channels with poorly developed elastica and muscularis, may be focal or diffuse and contain gross or microfistulae. Intranidal aneurysms may also be found. Venous features may include venous aneurysms, ectasia and stenoses (Lasjaunias et al., 1986; Lasjaunias & Berenstein, 1992). Aneurysms on pedicle feeding arteries and within the nidus are known to be risk factors for haemorrhage (Graf et al., 1983). Conversely, feeding vessel aneurysms may regress following embolisation of the AVM (Lasjaunias et al., 1988). The diagnostic angiogram thus defines the angioarchitecture of the lesion and, following multidisciplinary consultation, leads to selection of the appropriate treatment.

Preparation

In no other area of interventional neuroradiology is a team approach more important than in the treatment of AVMs. In particular, an experienced assistant is imperative. An understanding of the development, natural history and haemodynamics of these complex lesions is also a prerequisite. A decision should be made to aim for either complete obliteration at a single session or staged embolisation at multiple sessions. Informed consent is obtained and preoperative studies performed as described above. Endovascular treatment of AVMs is usually performed under light sedation. We do not routinely heparinise patients for this procedure.

Technique

Introducer sheaths and guiding catheters are inserted into the appropriate vessels as described previously. Embolisation with NBCA may be performed via flow-directed microcatheters or via catheter/guidewire combinations. In general, flow-directed catheters are more suitable for more distal, and especially high-flow, lesions. The catheter is navigated into the feeding vessel selected using roadmapping as required. Careful insertion of a guidewire into the proximal part of the flow-directed microcatheter may sometimes be useful, and cross compression of the opposite carotid artery can aid catheterisation of anterior cerebral vessels. Superselective angiograms are performed to identify the part of the nidus supplied by the vessel and any cortical branches. The flow-rate through that part of the AVM can also be assessed, and the volume of the nidus estimated, if desired. When the microcatheter is satisfactorily positioned close to, or in, the nidus and beyond any branches to normal brain, the NBCA mixture is prepared (see previous discussion) The microcatheter is flushed with 5% dextrose solution to prevent premature polymerisation. The NBCA adhesive is then injected under fluoroscopy over several seconds. As the injection is completed the neuroradiologist gives a pre-arranged signal at which the assistant smartly withdraws the microcatheter. This maneouvre clearly requires rehearsal and an alert assistant. Some workers recommend withdrawing the guiding catheter together with the microcatheter following each glue injection. An alternative technique requires wedging of the microcatheter in the nidus itself and prolonged injection of more dilute (20-30%) NBCA over 1-2 minutes in an attempt to completely fill the nidus (Debrun et al., 1997). Following the injection a repeat angiogram is performed to determine the need for further embolisation (Figure 2.8). Other pedicles may now be selected and embolised.

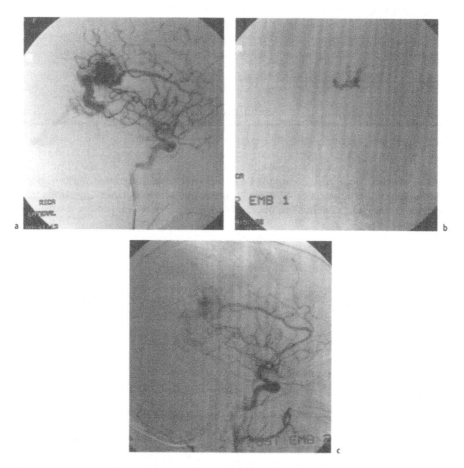

Fig. 2.8. Angiogram in this young woman presenting with intracerebral haemorrhage demonstrated a deep AVM located close to the splenium of the corpus callosum with venous drainage into the vein of Galen. Arterial supply was from the pericallosal artery **a**. Angiogram during injection of NBCA glue with flow-guided microcatheter at the nidus **b**. Almost complete occlusion of the nidus after two injections **c**.

Following completion of the procedure and post-embolisation angiograms, the guiding catheter and introducer sheath are removed as previously described.

Special Techniques for Arteriovenous Fistulae

The technique of embolisation may have to be modified for certain types of AVM. The very high flow-rate in an arteriovenous fistula (AVF) may make glue injections ineffective. In such cases neat NBCA glue may be injected in the pedicle if a sufficient safe length of vessel is available. If the glue is used without any dilution fluoroscopy is unnecessary during injection. Alternatively, reduced amounts of lipiodol or tungsten powder can be added. The use of detachable balloons may be appropriate in some AVFs. The balloon can be easily floated to the desired position and then fully inflated, which can result in complete treatment of the AVF (Figure 2.9). More recently, detachable microcoils have been used for some AVFs. Coils larger than the size of the fistula prevent their inadvertent embolisation into the venous side of the circulation.

Liquid coils (Bernstein coils) may also be used in such situation. They can be placed proximal to the fistula and can act as a focus for glue polymerisation

Peroperative Angiography

Peroperative angiography is a useful guide for the surgeon during excision of the AVM which commonly follows staged embolisation. It helps to localise a residual lesion and to assess complete excision. We usually place a 5F catheter, continuously perfused by a pressure bag containing 1000 u heparin in 1000 ml saline, in the main supplying vessel (usually common carotid artery) for the duration of the operation. After positioning the head for surgery, contrast medium injections allow identification of the AVM by image intensifier. Further injections can be made as needed during the operation. We use this technique for most large AVMs.

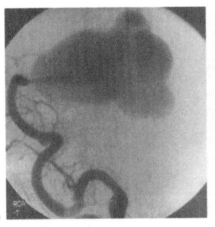 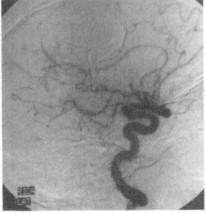

Fig. 2.9. An intracerebral arteriovenous fistula filling a giant venous varix **a**. This was occluded by a detachable balloon visible in **b**.

Complications

General complications are as for aneurysm embolisation (Berenstein et al., 1989). The major morbidity of AVM embolisation arises from embolism or inadvertent glue occlusion of normal vessels. Passage of glue through the AVM may result in pulmonary embolism. Delay in withdrawing the microcatheter following injection of adhesive may result in the catheter being glued permanently in place with the consequent risk of thromboembolism (Inci et al., 1996). Premature withdrawal, while the NBCA injection is in progress may be more disastrous, and will result in glue entering branches to normal brain.

Conclusion

The last 10 years have seen considerable advances in interventional techniques. These have resulted in an improved ability to treat many vascular lesions in the head safely and effectively. Although the basic techniques of endovascular access will probably remain unchanged for some time to come, the continuing development of new devices (including catheters, coils, stents and liquid embolic agents) is likely to change the specific procedures for treatment of intracranial aneurysms and AVMs. Improved techniques will also bring pressures to maintain good clinical practice and to offer better training programmes and facilities.

References

Alksne JF, Fingerhut AG (1965) Magnetically controlled metallic thrombosis of intracranial aneurysms. A preliminary report. Bull Los Angeles Neurolog Soc 30: 153-155

Aspoas AR, Gholkar A, Sengupta RP (1993) Peroperative vertebral arterial catheterisation for proximal control in aneurysm surgery. Br Neurosurg 7: 71-74

Berenstein A, Choi JS, Kupersmith M et al. (1989) Complications of endovascular embolisation in 182 patients with cerebral AVMs. AJNR 57: 7-10

Brothers MF, Kaufmann JCE, Fox AJ, Deveikis JP (1989) N-Butyl-2-cyanoacrylate: substitute for IBCA in interventional neuroradiology - histopathologic and polymerization time studies. AJNR 10: 777-786

Clouston JE, Numaguchi Y, Zoarski GH, Aldrich EF, Simard JM, Zitnay KM (1995) Intraarterial papaverine infusion for cerebral vasospasm after subarachnoid haemorrhage. AJNR 16: 27-38

Debrun GM, Aletich V, Ausman JI et al. (1997) Embolization of the nidus of brain arteriovenous malformations with n-butyl cyanoacrylate. Neurosurgery 40: 112-121

Dion JE, Duckwiler GR, Lylyk P et al. (1989) Progressive suppleness pursil catheter : a new tool for superselective angiography and embolization. AJNR 10: 1068-1070

Dion J (1992) Principles and methodology. In: Vinuela F, Halbach VV, Dion JE. (eds) Interventional Neuroradiology. New York, pp 1-15

Eskridge JM, Newell DW, Winn RH (1994) Endovascular treatment of vasospasm. Neurol Surg Clin N Am 5 (3): 437-447

Gallagher JP (1964) Pilojection for intracranial aneurysms. J Neurosurg 21: 129-134

Goto K, Halbach VV, Hardin CW et al. (1988) Permanent inflation of detachable balloons with a low-viscosity, hydrophylic polymerising system. Radiology 169: 787-790

Graf CJ, Perret GE, Torner JC (1983) Bleeding from cerebral arteriovenous malformations as part of their natural history. J. Neurosurg 58: 331-337

Guglielmi G, Vinuela F, Dion J, Duckwiler G (1991a) Electrothrombosis of saccular aneurysms via endovascular approach. Part 1. Electrochemical basis, technique and experimental results. J Neurosurg 75: 1–7

Guglielmi G, Vinuela F, Dion J et al. (1991b) Electrothrombosis of saccular aneurysms via endovascular approach. Part 2. Preliminary clinical experience. J Neurosurg 75: 8–14

Hilal SK (1988) Synthetic fibre coated platinum coils successfully used for the endovascular treatment of arteriovenous malformations, aneurysms and direct arteriovenous fistulae of the central nervous system (abstract). Radiology 169(suppl): 28–32

Hodes JE, Aymard A, Gobin YP et al. (1991) Endovascular occlusion of intracranial vessels for curative treatment of unclippable aneurysms: report of 16 cases. J Neurosurg 75: 694–701

Hosobuchi Y (1979) Direct surgical treatment of giant intracranial aneurysms. J Neurosurg 51: 743–756

Inci S, Ozcan OE, Benli K, Saatci I (1996) Microsurgical removal of a free segment of microcatheter in the anterior circulation as a complication of embolization. Surg Neurol 46: 562–567

Kikuchi Y, Strother CM, Boyer M (1987) New catheter for endovascular interventional procedures. Radiology 165: 870–871

Lasjaunias P, Manelfe C, Chiu M (1986) Angiographic architecture of intracranial vascular malformations and fistulas–pretherapeutic aspects. Neurosurg Rev 9: 253–264

Lasjaunias P, Piske R, Terbrugge K, Willinsky R (1988) Cerebral arteriovenous malformations (CAVM) and associated arterial aneurysms (AA). Analysis of 101 CAVM cases, with 37 AA in 23 patients. Acta Neurochir (Wien) 91: 29–35

Lasjaunias P, Berenstein A (1992) Chapter 1, Classification of brain arteriovenous malformations. In: Surgical neuroangiography, vol 4: Endovascular treatment of cerebral lesions. Berlin, Springer-Verlag, pp 25–80.

Luessenhop AJ, Spence WT (1960) Artificial embolization of cerebral arteries. Report of use in a case of arteriovenous malformation. JAMA 172: 1153–1155

Luessenhop AJ, Velasquez AC (1964) Observations on the tolerance of intracranial arteries to catheterisation. J Neurosurg 21: 85–91

Marks MP, Chee H, Liddell RP et al. (1994) A mechanically detachable coil for the treatment of aneurysms and occlusion of blood vessels. AJNR 15: 821–827

Marks MP, Steinberg GK, Lane B (1995) Combined use of endovascular coils and surgical clipping for intracranial aneurysms. AJNR 16: 15–18

Moret JG, Boulin A, Mawad ME, Castaings L (1993) Adjustable and detachable tungsten Spirales (MDS system) for treatment of intracranial aneurysms: characteristics of the device, comparison with existing detachable coils, analysis of results (Abstract). Am Soc Neuroradiol, 31st Annual Meeting, Vancouver, Canada

Moret J, Cognard C, Weill A et al. (1997) The "remodelling technique" in the treatment of wide neck intracranial aneurysms. Angiographic results and clinical follow-up in 56 cases. Intervent Neuroradiol 3: 21–35

Mullan S (1974) Experiences with surgical thrombosis of intracranial berry aneurysms and carotid cavernous fistulas. J Neurosurg 41: 657–670

Putman CM, Chaloupka JC (1996) Use of large-caliber coronary guiding catheters for neurointerventional applications. AJNR 17: 697–704

Serbinenko FA (1974) Balloon catheterisation and occlusion of major cerebral vessels. J Neurosurg 41: 125–145

Spetzler RF, Martin NA (1986) A proposed scheme for grading intracranial arteriovenous malformations. J Neurosurg 65: 476–483

Wikholm G (1995) Occlusion of cerebral arteriovenous malformations with N-butyl cyanoacrylate is permanent. AJNR 16: 479–482

Chapter 3

Endovascular Treatment of Intracranial Aneurysms: the Oxford Experience

W.E.H. Lim and James V. Byrne

Introduction

Rupture of intracranial berry aneurysms is the commonest cause of non-traumatic subarachnoid haemorrhage (SAH), with 10 to 15 new cases per 100 000 per annum in the United Kingdom (Brewis et al., 1966). The consequences of aneurysmal subarachnoid haemorrhage are mortality rates of 30–40% and rebleed rates of up to 29% in the first 3 weeks (Locksley, 1966). If untreated, up to 50% of ruptured aneurysms will rebleed in the first 6 months (Jane et al., 1985). The long-term outcome is also poor with only 36–50% of patients with aneurysmal SAH surviving with good outcome, i.e. Glasgow Outcome Scale (GOS) 4 or 5 (Jennet & Bond, 1975; Edner et al., 1992).

Traditionally, ruptured intracranial saccular aneurysms are treated surgically either by (i) procedures that occlude the aneurysm together with the parent vessel or (ii) procedures that obliterate the aneurysm and preserve flow within the parent vessel, by for example, placing a clip across its neck. For the past two decades, the endovascular approach has been developed to treat aneurysms, primarily as an alternative to surgery for complex aneurysms and for patients in which surgery or general anaesthesia were contraindicated. Initially, detachable balloons were used to occlude the parent artery (Serbinenko, 1974; Debrun et al., 1981) or obliterate the aneurysm with preservation of the parent artery (i.e. endosaccular packing) (Higashida et al., 1990a). Thrombogenic microcoils placed within the aneurysm sac have also been employed with good results (Hilal, 1990; Casasco et al., 1993). More recently, electrically detachable coils (GDC) (Guglielmi et al., 1991b) and mechanically detached coils (MDS) (Pierot et al., 1996) have been used. The GDC system, by virtue of its electrolytic detachment, allows for the controlled and precise placement of soft platinum coils within the aneurysm lumen (Gugliemi et al., 1991a). These devices have reduced the incidence of procedural complication and increased the range of aneurysms that can be treated by endovascular techniques.

Aims of Treatment

The objective of all types of surgical treatments for intracranial aneurysms is to prevent their rupture or growth. Most patients present with symptoms and signs due to aneurysm enlargement or rupture. In the setting of acute aneurysmal subarachnoid haemorrhage, the main aim of treatment, whether surgical or endovascular is to prevent, with the minimum of additional trauma, a potentially fatal rebleed. Furthermore by securing the aneurysm clinically symptomatic vasospasm, which is a major cause of morbidity and mortality in patients after SAH, can be more aggressively managed (Kassel et al., 1990a).

The goal of treatment for aneurysms presenting with mass effect is to relieve pressure on local neural structures and prevent their enlargement. Endoscaccular treatment is effective in relieving clinical symptoms because local pressure due to pulsation is reduced once flow within the aneurysm lumen ceases. Van Halbach reported complete resolution of neurological signs due to mass effect after treatment by endosaccular packing with balloons or coils in 50% and objective improvement in 42.3%, of a group of 26 patients (Van Halbach et al., 1994). They postulated that the response to treatment by endosaccular packing was due to both a decrease in aneurysm size as well as reduced transmitted arterial pulsation against adjacent structures once the aneurysm thrombosed.

Finally, aneurysms may be discovered incidentally during investigations for other reasons or coincidental to SAH in patients with multiple aneurysms. When considering treatment options for unruptured aneurysms, one must consider the natural history. The annual risk of haemorrhage has been estimated at approximately 1% (Juvela et al., 1993) and even lower by a large prospective study in which a rupture rate of 0.5% per annum was reported for aneurysms over 10 mm in size and only 0.05% per annum for smaller aneurysms (ISUIA investigators, 1998). The procedural risks of treatment related morbidity from surgery (Solomon et al., 1994) or endovascular therapy (Guglielmi et al., 1992) has been reported to be about 5% and therefore approximates to the untreated risk of bleeding over 5–10 years. In our institution, the decision to treat an incidental aneurysm by either route is made jointly with the patient after a thorough discussion of the specific risk and benefits.

Ideally, treatment to render the aneurysm harmless should preserve blood flow within the parent artery. In most cases simply isolating the aneurysm from the parent vessel by endosaccular packing or clipping of the neck is adequate. Unfortunately, some aneurysms by nature of their location and anatomy are best managed with parent artery (PA) occlusion. Surgically, this may be achieved by Hunterian ligation, i.e. occluding the parent artery proximal to the aneurysm neck or by trapping the aneurysm between proximal and distal arterial ligations (Steinburg et al., 1993; Drake et al., 1994). Endovascular techniques have now largely replaced extravascular surgery to achieve the same result (Fox et al., 1987; Aymard et al., 1991; Hodes et al., 1991). Both surgical and endovascular techniques may be supplemented by prior revascularization (bypass) surgery in order to maintain adequate cerebral blood flow after occlusion of the aneurysm bearing cranial arteries (Lawton et al., 1996).

Parent Artery Occlusion

Indications

Sacrifice of the parent artery for the treatment of intracranial aneurysms is indicated in the following situations:

Endovascular Treatment of Intracranial Aneurysms

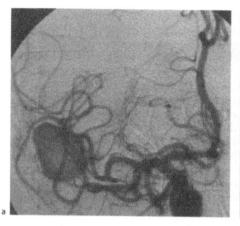
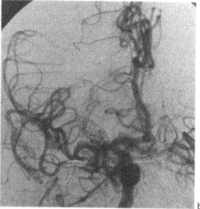

Fig. 3.1. Large, 16-mm diameter incidental aneurysm with a wide neck located at the origin of the inferior division, right middle cerebral artery **a**. It was felt that endosaccular packing would result in herniation of the coils and obstruction of the parent artery. Proximal occlusion of the parent artery with GDC and fibre coils was performed after balloon test occlusion demonstrated presence of good collateral support. The patient tolerated the procedure without development of any neurological deficits and there was no residual filling of the aneurysm on the control angiogram at 2 months **b**.

1. Giant saccular aneurysms (diameter greater than 25 mm), with wide necks and heavily calcified walls. These aneurysms are challenging problems for both conventional and endovascular surgery. For the endovascular therapist it may be difficult to visualise the aneurysm neck because it is often obscured by the large aneurysm sac, while the thickness of the wall, which may also be calcified and rigid hinders the extravascular surgeon, making it difficult to apply clips. In our experience, endosaccular coil packing of giant aneurysms is also associated with a high chance of recurrence, with aneurysm regrowth in 9 of 11 (80%) aneurysms on follow-up angiogram performed at 6 months (Byrne et al., 1996).
2. Ectatic, wide necked or fusiform aneurysms assessed to be unsuitable for clipping or endosaccular coil packing. Either because adjacent vessels have become incorporated into the neck of the aneurysm, or the configuration of the neck precludes stable deployment of coils (see Figure 3.1).
3. Small distal aneurysms, i.e. aneurysms arising at branch arteries distal to the circle of Willis. They may be difficult to locate during surgery and the small calibre of the parent vessel hinders endosaccular treatment. Collateral support in this distal location is usually satisfactory and its adequacy may be confirmed by functional testing with selective intra-arterial injection of sodium amytal.
4. Post-traumatic pseudoaneurysms and intracranial mycotic aneurysms which have fragile walls. The latter may occur on distal arteries and when collateral circulation is adequate, the endovascular route utilising balloons, acrylate glue or microcoils to occlude the PA and the aneurysm is efficacious and avoids surgery in ill patients (Scotti et al., 1996).

Technique

Generally, it is our practice to employ the endovascular route first for all patients as it offers the opportunity of testing the adequacy of collateral support by preliminary temporary test occlusion. This is performed with the patient anticoagulated and awake in order to be accessible for continuous neurological assessment. A balloon is placed at the proposed site of arterial occlusion and inflated for 20 minutes. Collateral flow is assessed periodically by angiography and may be supplemented by cerebral blood flow analysis employing stable xenon CT (Mathis et al., 1995) or SPECT (Peterman et al., 1991). Provocative testing with hypotensive challenge has also been advocated to increase the sensitivity of the test in light of the up to 22% rate of false negative test occlusions (Standard et al., 1995). Using a detachable balloon for the test, immediate balloon deployment can be implemented if collateral supply is adequate. This technique minimises the theoretical risk of emboli arising upon balloon deflation, from the static columns of blood proximal and distal to the occlusion balloon. If the aneurysm has recently ruptured, the procedure is usually delayed for 4–6 weeks, to allow the patient to recover from the effects of the SAH (such as vasospasm), thus decreasing the risk of ischaemic complications.

Results and Complications

The results of endovascular and surgical PA occlusion for the treatment of intracranial aneurysms are summarised in Table 3.1. The efficacy of treatment is related to the likelihood of retrograde filling of the aneurysm (see Figure 3.2). In the series of Fox et al. there was a marked reduction in successful obliteration of aneurysms located at or above the origin of the ophthalmic artery (Fox et al., 1987). This low obliteration rate compared to infraclinoid aneurysms is presumably due to filling of the aneurysm via the circle of Willis or through external carotid to internal carotid artery (e.g. ophthalmic artery) collaterals. Fox also reported a 12.3% incidence (eight patients) of delayed ischaemia post occlusion, which responded to treatment by volume expansion, heparin and aspirin and one case of permanent neurological deficit in a series of 65 treated patients.

Table 3.1. Parent artery occlusion: treatment results

Series author and aneurysm site	No. of cases	Complete thrombosis (%)	Rebleeding rates	Morbidity	Mortality
Fox et al., 1987 (endovascular) $n = 65$					
Carotid artery below ophthalmic artery	37	100	none reported	13.2% (9 cases) (1.5% permanent, 12.3% transient)	nil
Carotid artery at or above ophthalmic artery	21	50			
Basilar artery with VA occlusion	6	50			
Vertebral artery	1	100			
Steinberg et al., 1993 (surgery) $n = 201$					
Vertebral artery	36	89*	6% (12 cases at 1 week post surgery)	25% (50 cases including 6% who rebled & 2.5% with vasospasm)	12% at 1 month 19.5% at 1 year 24% long term (cumulative)
Vertebrobasilar junction	35	86*			
Basilar trunk	46	89*			
Basilar bifurcation	83	65*			
Aymard et al., 1991 (endovascular) $n = 21$					
Vertebrobasilar	21	62	5% (1 of 21 cases) patient later died	10% (2 cases, including 1 who rebled)	5% procedure-related 10% total

* Also includes virtually complete thrombosis.

Endovascular Treatment of Intracranial Aneurysms

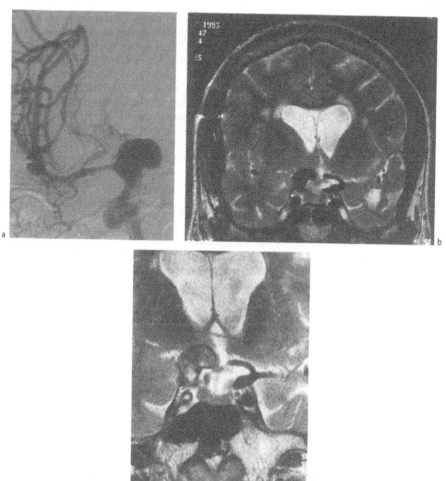

Fig. 3.2. ICA angiogram demonstrating a large wide necked right internal carotid artery termination aneurysm in a patient who presented with subarachnoid haemorrhage **a**. It was explored at craniotomy, deemed to be unclippable and treated by wrapping. The aneurysm was managed endovascularly by proximal occlusion of the right ICA below the level of the ophthalmic artery since during test occlusion, only minimal cross flow via the anterior communication artery was demonstrated. Pre-treatment T2 weighted coronal MRI records flow void within the lumen of the aneurysm **b**. Follow-up MRI study at 2 months shows high signal representing thrombosis within the right ICA and the aneurysm lumen **c**.

Drake et al. (1994) reported similar occlusion rates for supraclinoid aneurysms in their series of 160 giant carotid artery aneurysms treated by PA occlusion or aneurysm trapping. They were able to confirm complete aneurysm occlusion in 11 of 23 (49%) ophthalmic and paraophthalmic aneurysms, and 4 of 7 (57%) posterior communicating aneurysms. Complete occlusion was established in 17 of 21 (80%) carotid bifurcation aneurysms, with 10 of the cases requiring intracranial occlusion, trapping or occlusion of the A1 segment of the anterior communicating artery to achieve complete treatment. Clinical outcome was reported to be excellent or good in 44 of 51 cases (86%).

In the posterior circulation, Steinberg et al. (1993) achieved successful aneurysm thrombosis in 78% of his total cohort using surgical techniques, with excellent or good clinical results in 73%. Aymard et al. (1991) established angiographic cure in 13 of 21 patients managed via the endovascular route, with 67% of the patients returning to normal function.

Rebleed rates for both surgical (Steinberg et al., 1993) and endovascular (Aymard et al., 1991) parent artery occlusion for unclippable posterior circulation aneurysms appear to be similar, with a longer mean follow up period in the surgical group of 9.5 years versus 2 years after endovascular treatment (Table 3.1). Morbidity at one month, reported by Steinberg, was due to direct surgical trauma in 3.5%, to vertebrobasilar ischaemia resulting in permanent deficits in 13% and from early rebleeding after treatment in 6%, giving a total treatment related morbidity rate of 22.5%. Although the two series are not directly comparable because of the patients selected for treatment, the morbidity figure for the surgical series is double the treatment related morbidity of Aymard's admittedly smaller cohort.

A possible late complication of PA occlusion procedures is de novo aneurysm formation and/or enlargement (Tiperman et al., 1995). The risk however appears to be small and does not deter us from performing PA sacrifice, given that it is often the only therapeutic option available for complex aneurysms (Boardman and Byrne, 1998).

Therefore, both surgical and endovascular routes appear to be equally effective methods of inducing aneurysm thrombosis, but because of the safety afforded by test occlusion in the awake patient and lower perioperative morbidity, the endovascular route offers significant advantages.

Table 3.2. Oxford treatment protocol for endovascular coil embolisation

Pre-procedure
- Indications and therapeutic options reviewed with neurosurgeon
- Informed consent
- Aspirin/antiplatelet agents for wide necked aneurysms; withheld in acutely ruptured aneurysms

Procedure
- General anaesthesia preferred
- Systemic anti-coagulation (5000 iu of heparin sodium as an i.v. bolus plus hourly increments of 1000–2000 iu to maintain coagulation two to three times baseline activated thromboplastin time), unless contraindicated. Initial dose is administered prior to guide catheter placement
- Working angiographic projection selected to give best view of aneurysm neck
- Aneurysm catheterised with suitably shaped microcatheter
- Coil selected and deployed under fluroscopic 'roadmap' guidance
- Coil position within aneurysm and patency of parent vessel confirmed angiographically prior to coil detachment
- Further coils placed to fill aneurysm sac and occlude in-flow
- Post treatment control angiograms to document aneurysm occlusion and patency of adjacent vessels

Post procedure
- Heparin continued for 12 to 24 hours (between 500 to 1000 iu i.v. per hour) unless contraindicated
- Close clinical monitoring for complications
- Control angiogram at 6 months for all patients, or sooner if subtotal occlusion obtained

Endosaccular Packing

Endosaccular packing techniques have continued to evolve rapidly over the last decade. Intra-aneurysmal balloons have been superseded by detachable coils and more recently, controlled detachable coils. The goal of endosaccular packing is to isolate the aneurysm sac from the parent artery by occlusion of the aneurysm inflow and thus induce intra-aneurysmal thrombosis.

Since 1992, over 700 patients with cranial aneurysms have been treated with Guglielmi detachable coils (GDC, Target Therapeutics, Freemont USA) at Oxford. The initial results in ruptured and surgically unclippable aneurysms (Byrne et al., 1995a, b) as well as posterior fossa aneurysms (Molyneux et al., 1995) have been encouraging and the endovascular route with GDC is now used in the treatment of most infratentorial aneurysms.

Selection Criteria for Endovascular Treatment

Patient selection criteria for any given treatment modality are dependant on the technical feasibility and limitations of the treatment, as well as its effectiveness. These factors will vary from centre to centre, based on the locally available expertise and resources. The final decision regarding treatment in an individual patient should be a joint decision between the neurosurgeon, the endovascular therapist and the neuroanaesthetist. We have elected to review the selection criteria for coil embolisation of intracranial saccular aneurysms by considering them as (a) anatomical and (b) clinical criteria.

The necessary anatomical information can usually be ascertained from intra-arterial angiography supplement by axial computed tomography (CT) and/or magnetic resonance imaging (MRI) studies. Occasionally, when there is doubt, CT angiography (CTA) or MR angiography (MRA) with 3D surface rendering may yield additional detail and aid in pre-treatment assessment.

Anatomical Considerations

Access Tortuous proximal vasculature at the aortic arch and great vessels may defeat attempts at selective and stable catheterization of the internal carotid (ICA) or vertebral (VA) arteries for guide catheter placement. This is an uncommon problem given the hydrophilic guidewire and catheter systems presently available. However, it is occasionally necessary to percutaneously puncture the supra-aortic arteries in order to obtain endovascular access. Tortuous intracranial arteries with acute angulation of vessels at bifurcation points may hinder microcatheter navigation and increase the risk of catheter kinking, which impedes coil delivery or retrieval.

The endovascular route may be preferred because surgical access for certain intracranial aneurysms may also be limited by their location (e.g. basilar artery and paraophthalmic aneurysms), or when there has been contralateral brain surgery, for example in patients with multiple aneurysms, in order to avoid bilateral craniotomy.

Location The location of an aneurysm also has a bearing on the procedural risk and the treatment results of both endovascular and extravascular treatments. As stated previously, at our institution, most posterior fossa aneurysms are treated via the endovascular route, because of the relatively easy access and low procedural risks we have experienced. For anterior circulation aneurysms extravascular access is easier and the relative risk of the two approaches are similar. To resolve this issue, we are currently conducting a randomised multicenter trial comparing outcome in patients treated by surgical clipping or GDC for acutely ruptured aneurysms when it is judged, on current data, that clinical equipoise exists between the two treatments. More definite recommendations on the appropriateness of treatments, according to aneurysm locations can be made once the results become available.

Aneurysm Size Aneurysms smaller than or equal to 2 mm cannot be treated with GDC as the smallest coil currently available is 2 mm in diameter. Realistically we would prefer to limit endosaccular packing to aneurysms with a minimum diameter of 3 mm or greater.

The actual sac diameter of an aneurysm also affects the degree of occlusion that is attainable. In a series of the first 199 patients treated at Oxford, total occlusion was obtained in 72% of small (<10 mm), 61% of large (10-25 mm) and in 48% of giant aneurysm (Byrne et al., 1996). This relationship between the degree of occlusion and aneurysm size is similar to Casasco et al.'s experience with fibre coils (Casasco et al., 1993) where the complete occlusion rates were 94%, 82% and 60% and Vinuele et al. who reported rates of 70.8%, 35% and 50% (Vinuele et al., 1997) for correspondingly sized aneurysms.

Aneurysm Neck Anatomy The relationship of the aneurysm neck with the adjacent vessels must be clearly demonstrated in order to avoid coils herniating into the parent or adjacent arteries. The aneurysm neck should be discrete and must not incorporate any of the adjacent vessels. Superselective injection through the microcatheter may aid in demonstrating the requisite detail. Failure to ascertain the exact vascular relationships at the aneurysm site is a contraindication to endosaccular coil occlusion and most of the difficulties we have encountered in regard to visualisation of aneurysm neck anatomy have been with middle cerebral artery bifurcation aneurysms where adjacent branch arteries may overlap the neck region.

Neck Diameter An absolute neck diameter of more than 4 mm (classified as wide neck) has been showed to be associated with a lower rate of complete aneurysm occlusion. Zubillaga, demonstrated a 85% success rate at follow-up for aneurysms with necks ≤4 mm compared with only 15.7% where the neck was >4 mm (Zubillaga et al., 1994). This is because in wide necked aneurysms, it is often difficult to attain a dense pack of coils across the neck, due to the greater risk (c.f. small neck aneurysms) of coil herniation and migration into the parent vessel. In our patients the best long-term angiographic results were obtained in aneurysms that were initially densely packed, and/or had a narrow neck (Hope et al., 1999).

Neck/Size Ratio The diameter of the aneurysm neck relative to the aneurysm sac has also been used to discriminate between aneurysms suitable and unsuitable for endosaccular packing. The neck diameter and the largest sac diameter is easily obtained from the angiograms or CTA. A neck to sac size (N/S) ratio of <1:3 is deemed to be favourable for GDC treatment while it would be almost impossible to occlude completely one with a ratio of >1:1 (see Figure 3.3) without a significant risk of coil migration, coil prolapse or occlusion of the parent vessel. For N/S ratios >1:3 and <1:1, complete occlusion may be more difficult to achieve, and often small neck remnants have to be accepted. The use of a helper balloon positioned in the parent artery reduces the risk of herniation or migration of endosaccular coils

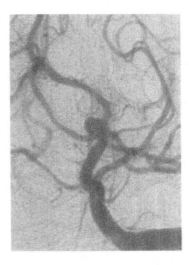

Fig. 3.3. Small but wide necked aneurysm arising from the origin of the right middle cerebral artery with a aneurysm neck to sac ratio of >1:1. Endovascular exploration was carried out but treatment could not be implemented due to herniation of coil loops into the parent vessel.

(Moret et al., 1997) and may allow the treatment of aneurysms with unfavourable ratios.

Wall Thickness Aneurysms with thick walls or wall calcification can make surgical clipping difficult but they do not hinder coil deployment and empirically may even be beneficial, by decreasing the risk of coil perforation. However, thick-walled aneurysms are frequently lined by soft thrombus, into which coils may compact, increasing the likelihood of recurrence.

Presence of Haematoma Cerebral parenchymal haematomas associated with aneurysm rupture may be small and, therefore, not require surgical evacuation. They are then not a contraindication to embolisation, and in fact, the endovascular route may be advantageous as it minimises operative trauma to the brain. When the haematoma requires evacuation, a combined approach with the aneurysm being secured with coils prior to surgery is an alternative we sometimes employ in poor grade patients so that surgery can be confined to haematoma evacuation.

Vasospasm Angiographic spasm by itself is not a contraindication to endovascular treatment, although when severe, it may restrict microcatheter entry to the aneurysm. In such instances, intra-arterial papaverine is infused via the microcatheter to dilate proximal vessels and to improve access. The risk that catheterization itself will aggravate arterial vasospasm is probably minimal (Rowe et al., 1995) and early endovascular treatment, by securing the aneurysm against rerupture allows patients to be treated by measures that increase cerebral blood flow. Surgery, on the other hand, is generally contraindicated when there is severe symptomatic or angiographic vasospasm (Kassel et al., 1990b).

Intra-aneurysmal Clot The presence of a significant amount of soft, acute intra-aneurysmal thrombus is a relative contraindication to coil treatment since it increases the risk of thromboembolic complications, delayed coil compaction and aneurysm regrowth. Early follow up is recommended in such patients (see above).

Amount of Subarachnoid Blood The severity of vasospasm has been shown to correlate with the volume and the duration of haemorrhage in the subarachnoid space (Fisher et al., 1980). Based on this observation, cisternal rinsing and lysis of clot with fibrinolytic agents has been advocated by some centres in order to reduce the risk of delayed cerebral vasospasm which may be used as a factor for selecting patients for craniotomy and clipping. However, the only randomised trial employing recombinant tissue plasminogen activator (Findlay et al., 1995), concluded that while the severity of angiographic vasospasm is reduced in patients with thick clots, there was no significant effect on symptomatic vasospasm. We feel that based on current knowledge, the benefit of cisternal rinsing is uncertain and the amount of subarachnoid clot does not influence our treatment selection.

Clinical Considerations

Clinical Grade The clinical grade of the patient on admission to hospital after SAH is generally scored on the Hunt and Hess (HH) or World Federation of Neurological Surgeons (WFNS) scales (Hunt & Hess, 1968; Drake, 1988) and is an important prognostic indicator of outcome. The majority of patients with good HH grades (Grades I and II) will have equally favourable outcomes with early surgical or endovascular treatments (Edner et al., 1992; Byrne et al., 1995). While a moderate or poor HH grade (III, IV and V) is considered to be a relative contraindication to early surgery; it is our current policy to offer coil embolisation to such patients in the hope that the minimally invasive approach improves clinical outcomes.

Age and Associated Medical Conditions Increased patient age on its own (>65 years) has been shown to be associated with a poorer overall management outcome in surgically treated patients (Kassel et al., 1990b). Therefore, in elderly patients or patients with medical conditions that significantly increase surgical and anaesthetic risks (e.g. ischaemic heart disease) endovascular coil occlusion is preferred (Rowe et al., 1996).

Timing of Therapy Timing of aneurysm surgery remains controversial. The International Co-operative Study on the Timing of Aneurysm Surgery (Kassel et al., 1990 a, b) concluded that there was no significant difference in management outcome in patients treated with either early or late surgery. It clearly demonstrated that the incidence of surgical complications was highest when surgery was performed during the intermediate periods: day 7-10 (10%) and days 4-6 (7.7%) compared with 5.5% when surgery was delayed until 11 days or later after SAH. Thus, it appears that the benefit of preventing rebleeding with early surgery is offset by the higher surgical morbidity incurred.

In our experience, timing of endosaccular coiling is less restricted by the interval between ictus and treatment. However, to obtain maximum benefit from the prevention of morbidity due to rebleeding, treatment should be carried out as soon as possible after the diagnosis of aneurysm rupture.

History of Previous Subarachnoid Haemorrhage or Surgery A history of multiple SAH or previous surgery may make the surgical approach to the aneurysm more difficult due to the formation of adhesions and scar tissue. Conversely, these conditions do not restrict endovascular methods.

Technique

Our standard protocol for endosaccular packing with the GDC system is listed in Table 3.2. Some of the more practical issues regarding technique will be discussed.

Coil and Catheter Selection

For small acutely ruptured aneurysms with fragile walls, the GDC-10 system of coils or the newly introduced "soft coils" are preferred as they deform more easily and cause less distortion of the aneurysm sac. The GDC-18 coils are used for larger aneurysms where softness of the coil is less of a concern and more coils are required for packing. In many instances, the standard 2 tip micro-catheters will suffice. Their higher friction may limit manoeuvrability in tortuous vessels, but it also endows greater stability to the system. Hydrophilic (FasTracker, Target Therapeutics, Freemont, USA) catheters on the other hand are more manoeuvrable but also more difficult to control. Catheter kinking is a problem when there are tortuous vessels but may be minimised by ensuring that the tension within the microcatheter system is kept low or by the use of braided kink-resistant catheters.

In order to select the correct helical coil diameter, the smallest diameter of the aneurysm lumen is measured from an angiogram corrected for magnification. The helical coil diameter chosen is slightly smaller (GDC-18) or just larger (GDC-10) than the aneurysm diameter.

Coil Packing

Most saccular aneurysms may be treated by using the initial coil to form a three-dimensional basket conforming to the shape of the aneurysm, with loops deployed across the neck of the aneurysm. This basket serves to contain the subsequent coils within the centre of the aneurysm. Smaller aneurysms may not avail themselves to this technique and one can treat these by deploying the coils to form a complex meshwork within the sac or use complex shaped coils such as 3D coils.

Complications of Endosaccular Coil Occlusion

Complications arising from endosaccular occlusion may be separated into those that are (a), immediate and, thus, most often related to the procedure or (b), delayed.

Immediate/Procedure-related Complications

The procedure-related complication rate of endosaccular coil occlusion varies between 9% and 15 %. Cassasco recorded two vascular perforations, four inadvertent PA occlusions and two embolic phenomena in his group of 71 patients treated with platinum microcoils; giving a rate of 11.3% (Casasco et al., 1993). In the multicentre study of Vinuela et al., (1997), 37 technical complications occurred in 403 treatments (9.18%). In this series of patients treated acutely after subarachnoid haemorrhage, perforation occurred in 2.7%, unintentional parent artery occlusion in 3% and thromboembolic events in 2.48% of patients.

Immediate complications encountered during endosaccular coil occlusion may be classified into three main groups: (i) haemorrhagic (ii) ischaemic (iii) technical.

Haemorrhagic Perforation of the aneurysm by the coil or microcatheter is usually immediately appreciated on angiography by the extravasation of contrast into the subarachnoid space. Initial management includes stopping all heparin containing infusions and reversing previously administered heparin with protamine sulphate. Additional coils are then deployed to seal the perforation. The majority of patients with small perforations do well when managed in this fashion. Both patients in Casasco's group and two of the three in our series (Byrne et al., 1995b) made good recovery. In contrast, bleeding may be more extensive and outcome poor when there is a large laceration, or when perforation occurs before deployment of the initial coil.

Aneurysm rupture and bleeding during induction of anaesthesia, craniotomy or dissection of the aneurysm neck can occur in 13 to 25% of patients treated surgically (Sundt et al., 1982; Edner et al., 1992). However, similar to endovascular treatment, most perforations do not result in permanent morbidity.

Ischaemic Procedure related ischaemic complication may be due either to thromboembolic phenomena or thrombosis of the PA and/or adjacent branch arteries.

Thromboemboli can arise from the guidecatheter, microcatheter or microguidewire, coils and from dislodged intra-aneurysmal clot. To prevent its occurrence, all patients are routinely anticoagulated during the procedure and catheters are constantly flushed with heparinised saline. When clinically possible, treatment should be avoided in the presence of fresh intra-aneurysmal thrombus, which might be dislodged by the microcatheter or coils.

Occlusion of parent or branch arteries may be secondary to herniation or prolapse of coils through the aneurysm neck, extension of intraluminal thrombosis or compression by the embolised aneurysm. If it occurs prior to coil detachment, the offending coil may be repositioned to restore normal flow. At times there is a delay before the vessel occludes. We therefore postpone coil detachment for a few minutes when we suspect that adjacent vessel integrity may be compromised, releasing the coil only when delayed angiography is satisfactory.

Arterial thrombosis may be treated by immediate administration of fibrinolytic drugs but we are concerned about the safety of intra-arterial thrombolysis performed after recent SAH and would prefer to support endogenous fibrinolysis by maintaining anticoagulation and perfusion. Prevention seems to be the key and one should avoid overpacking aneurysms, especially those with wide necks.

Technical Coil stretching can occur after repeated adjustment of the coil during deployment. It is suspected when (a) there is loss of the one-for-one response between coil movement and manipulation of the delivery wire or (b) a decrease in the radio-opacity of the coil at its junction zone as it begins to stretch. Other complications that can occur with coils include distal migration, breakage, and partial dislodgement into the PA. Coils that migrate can be recovered with various retriever devices. However, herniation of a short length of coil into the PA is no cause for alarm and is best managed by leaving it in situ, and maintaining anticoagulation and antiplatelet therapy for up to 2 months.

Arterial dissection and groin haematomas are other complications that may occur. Large haematomas can go unrecognised if they collect in the retroperitoneal space; if severe, the resultant anaemia and hypovolaemia may mimic symptoms of vasospasm or hydrocephalus and complicate patient management.

Delayed Complications

Delayed complications may either be due to the disease process or the treatment given, and it is often difficult to separate the effects of each group because of their similar clinical signs and symptoms.

Vasospasm/Delayed Ischaemic Deficit Angiographic vasospasm refers to the narrowing of vessel calibre that occurs after subarachnoid haemorrhage. It is seen in up to 67.3% of cases when angiography is performed between days 4 and 11 after SAH when it is most common. Half of these patients develop symptoms of cerebral ischaemia, i.e. symptomatic vasospasm; of these, a third die and another third are left with permanent neurological deficits (Dorsch, 1995).

There are a multitude of treatment regimes advocated for the prevention of post-SAH vasospasm and the treatment of symptomatic vasospasm. They include: (a) calcium channel antagonist drugs, of which nimodipine is the most commonly used; (b) a regime of induced hypertension/hypervolaemia/haemodilution, so-called triple H (H/H/H) therapy; (c) surgical lavage to remove subarachnoid clot; (d) endovascular treatments by angioplasty and intra-arterial infusions of papaverine. It is beyond the scope of this chapter to discuss in detail the first three therapies, suffice to say that that both nimodipine and H/H/H therapy can reduce the incidence and improve the outcome of vasospasm. The reader is directed to the excellent recent review of the subject by Dorsch (1995).

Transluminal balloon angioplasty (TLA) was initially utilised for the treatment of cerebral artery vasospasm induced during neurointerventional procedures and for patients with symptomatic post-subarachnoid haemorrhage vasospasm refractory to conventional therapies. The dilatation produced by successful angioplasty appears to be permanent although the exact mechanism is still unclear. Higashida et al. were able to restore normal vessel calibre in all 40 vascular territories treated by TLA, with immediate clinical improvement in 11 of 14 patients (79%) (Higashida et al., 1990b), while Newell et al. demonstrated sustained angiographic and neurological improvement in 8 of 10 patients with ischaemic symptoms after aneurysmal SAH. Six of the eight patients made good recovery while two were left with moderate disability (Newell et al., 1989). Taking into account the dire status of patients with intractable vasospasm, the results obtained in the above series are very encouraging, and support the use of TLA in this select group of patients.

Intra-arterial papaverine has also been advocated for the treatment of vasospasm (Kassel et al., 1992). However, as its effects are transient and of short duration, we prefer to rely on medical therapy or TLA for the management of symptomatic vasospasm and use papaverine when we require short term vasodilatation to improve access for aneurysm catheterisation or TLA.

Hydrocephalus Acute obstructive hydrocephalus diagnosed on axial imaging is a frequent occurrence after SAH. Hasan et al. reported an incidence of 21.5% (102 of 473 patients), of whom 75% were clinically symptomatic (Hasan et al., 1989). Communicating hydrocephalus may also be a complication in the subacute and late phase after SAH. Treatment is usually reserved for symptomatic patients and consists of external drainage in the acute stage and ventricular shunting if hydrocephalus persists. Serial lumbar cerebrospinal fluid taps or lumbar shunts may also help relieve the symptoms of communicating hydrocephalus.

Other Complications Other complications include late thromboembolic events, which may cause transient symptoms presumably due to thromboemboli generated from the surface of coils. Such symptoms may occur up to 6 weeks after coil embolisation and usually respond to treatment with low dose oral aspirin or warfarin (Byrne et al., 1995a).

Treatment Results

Before a new treatment is adopted, it must be shown to be as effective or better than current therapy and to be as safe or safer. The current best therapy for intracranial saccular aneurysms is surgical clipping, with which coil embolisation has to be compared.

The procedural morbidity and mortality figures presented in Table 3.3 demonstrate that endosaccular coil packing is a relatively safe technique. Reported morbidity rates are similar or lower than surgery in the patients treated with coils, despite the fact that most of these patients were considered unsuitable for surgical clipping or had failed surgery. Procedural mortality rates were fairly similar between the listed reports despite the differences in treatment types and selection criteria.

Endoscaccular coils have been shown to be effective in bringing about aneurysm occlusion in the short term (Table 3.3 and Figure 3.4). Its long-term stability, however, has been questioned, especially when it is employed in the treatment of large, wide-necked, or termination aneurysms. We have recently reported the first 465 patients referred for endosaccular coil treatment to the Radcliffe Infirmary (Byrne et al., 1999). Of this group, 317 patients were successfully treated within 30 days of SAH and have been followed up with a protocol which consists of a control angiogram and clinical assessment at 6 months (supplementary angiograms were performed when warranted) and a postal questionnaire annually. Delayed spontaneous subarachnoid haemorrhage occured in five patients, three within 18 months of treatment and two after 2 years.

Aneurysm regrowth was seen in 13.6% of small, 14.8% of large and 100% of giant aneurysms at 6 months. This appreciable percentage of regrowth in the small and

Table 3.3. Treatment of intracranial aneurysms – endovascular and surgical procedural morbidity and mortality

Series	Complete occlusion (%)	Incomplete occlusion (%)	Good recovery (%)	Morbidity (%)	Mortality (%)
Casasco et al., 1993 $n = 71$ (Endovascular fibre coils)	84.5	15.5	84.5 at 6 mths	4.2	7
Byrne et al., 1995 $n = 69$ (Endovascular GDC)	79	21	87 at 6 wks	7.2	2.8
Vinuela et al., 1997 $n = 403$ (Endovascular GDC)	50–70	30–50	Not given	8–9	6
Sundt et al., 1982 $n = 644$ (Surgical clipping, and PA occlusion)			72 at discharge	9.8	4.4
Edner et al., 1992 $n = 122$ (Surgical clipping)			62 at discharge 67 at 6 mths 69 at 1 yr	7.4	3.3
Guglielmi et al., 1992[†] $n = 42$ (Endovascular GDC)	42	58	86	4.8	2.4
Peerless et al., 1994[†] $n = 206$ (Surgical clipping, PA occlusions, and three cases endovascular)	87.4	12.6	84.2	8.5	6.5

† Series of vertebrobasilar aneurysms, GDC: Guglielmi detachable coils, PA: parent artery.

Endovascular Treatment of Intracranial Aneurysms

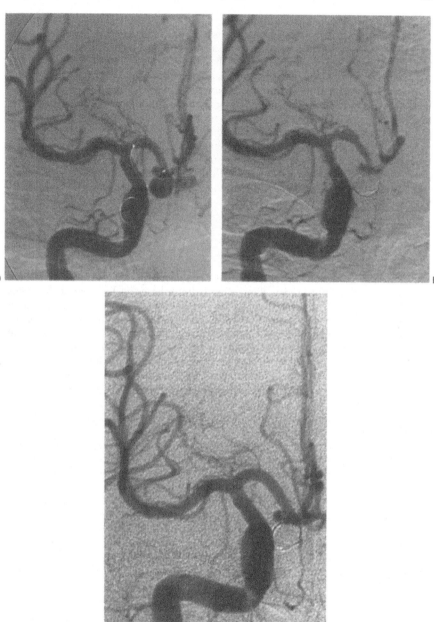

Fig. 3.4. Right anterior cerebral artery A1/A2 junction aneurysm in a 33 year woman who presented with subarachnoid haemorrhage **a**. Note the presence of the microcatheter tip just at the neck of the aneurysm. Immediate post procedure control shows complete occlusion of the aneurysm **b**, there is arterial spasm noted in the distal ICA and A1 segment of the anterior cerebral artery. The 6-month control angiogram **c** demonstrates stable occlusion with no evidence of aneurysm regrowth.

large aneurysms is of some concern and may be partially explained by our treatment philosophy for acutely ruptured aneurysms in poor grade patients. The aim of treatment in these instances was to achieve an acceptable degree of occlusion with minimal procedural morbidity, so that the risk of rebleeding was minimised and conditions for the management of complications made optimal. Should subsequent angiography demonstrate significant regrowth, further coils or surgery can then be used to complete treatment. A policy endorsed by the finding that unstable occlusion on 6 month angiography was associated with a 7.8% incidence of subsequent rebleeding compared with only 0.4% for stable occlusions (Byne et al., 1999).

The poor long-term occlusion of giant aneurysms reflects the complex problems that these aneurysms present. Unfortunately, surgery for giant aneurysms is also associated with poor outcomes. Faced with these limitations, we feel that coil treatment is often the best available option in the difficult situation when balloon occlusion of the PA or surgery are not feasible.

Summary

Endovascular methods for the treatment of intracranial aneurysm have evolved rapidly over the past 20 years. Pioneering balloon based technology of the 1970s introduced to the neuroscience world a minimally invasive method of dealing with a disease that has a high natural and treatment-related morbidity and mortality. When used to bring about parent vessel occlusion, endovascular balloons were not only effective, they were also relatively inexpensive and simple to use. However, they were less successful when endosaccular occlusion of the aneurysm was required. Since they did not conform to the shape of the aneurysm lumen, occlusion was frequently subtotal and aneurysm rupture occurred because they were more rigid than coils. Moreover, the complexities of exchanging radiographic contrast in the balloon with a solidifying agent meant that these procedures were usually only undertaken in a few specialised centres.

Since its introduction in 1990, the GDC system has revolutionalized the management of intracranial aneurysms, especially in poor grade patients and for surgically unsuitable aneurysms. Conceptually, it is an elegant technique, as it allows the therapist to resite the coil until a satisfactory position is obtained and then use nonmechanical electrolysis to achive detachment. Initial enthusiasm for the ability of the coil to bring about aneurysm occlusion has however, been tempered with midterm results that reveal a propensity for some aneurysms to regrow despite near complete initial occlusion. We are hopeful that ongoing research to improve coil thrombogenicity and stability may solve part of the regrowth problem and wait expectantly for the development of alternative endovascular techniques.

References

Aymard A, Gobin YP, Hodes JE et al. (1991) Endovascular occlusion of vertebral arteries in the treatment of unclippable vertebrobasilar aneurysms. J Neurosurg 74: 393–398

Boardman P, Byrne JV (1998) Giant fusiform basilar artery aneurysm: endovascular treatment by flow reversal in the basilar artery. British Journal of Radiology 71: 332–335

Brewis M, Poskanzer DC, Rolland C, Miller C (1966) Neurological disease in an English city. Acta Neurol Scand (suppl) 42(24): 1–89

Byrne JV, Adams CBT, Kerr RSC et al. (1995a) Endosaccular treatment of inoperable intracranial aneurysms with platinum coils. Br J Neurosurg 9: 585–592

Byrne JV, Molyneux AJ, Brennan RP, Renowden SA (1995b) Embolisation of recently ruptured intracranial aneurysms. Br J Neurosurg, Neurosurg & Psychiatr 59 S: 616–620

Byrne JV, Bacon F, Higgins N et al. (1996) Coil embolization of intracranial aneurysms: follow-up results. Proceedings of the 34th Annual Meeting, American Society of Neuroradiology, p 138

Byrne JV, Sohn MJ, Molyneux AJ (1999) Five-year experience in using coil embolization for ruptured intracranial aneurysms: outcomes and incidence of late rebleeding. Journal of Neurosurgery 90: 656–663

Casasco AE, Aymard A, Gobin P et al. (1993) Selective endovascular treatment of 71 intracranial aneurysms with platinum coils. J Neurosurg 79: 3–10

Debrun G, Fox A, Drake C et al. (1981) Giant unclippable aneurysms: treatment with detachable balloons. Am J Neuroradiol 2: 167–173

Dorsch NWC (1995) Cerebral arterial vasospasm – a clinical review. Br J Neurosurg 9: 403–412

Drake CG (1988) Report of World Federation of Neurological Surgeons Committee on a universal subarachnoid haemorrhage grading scale. J Neurosurg 68: 985–986

Drake CG, Peerless SJ, Ferguson GG (1994) Hunterian proximal arterial occlusion for giant aneurysms of the carotid circulation. J Neurosurg 81: 656–665

Edner G, Kagstroms E, Wallstedt L (1992) Total overall management and surgical outcome after aneurysmal subarachnoid haemorrhage in a defined population. Br J Neurosurg 6: 409–420

Fisher CM, Kistler JP, Davies JM (1980) Relation of cerebral vasospasm to subarachnoid hemorrhage, visualized by computerised tomographic scanning. Journal of Neurosurgery 6: 1–9

Fox AJ, Vinuela F, Pelz DM et al. (1987) Use of detachable balloon for proximal artery occlusion in the treatment of unclippable cerebral aneurysms. J Neurosurg 66: 40–46

Gugliemi G, Vinuela F, Sepetka I et al. (1991a) Electhrombosis of saccular aneurysms via endovascular approach. Part 1: Electrochemical basis, technique and experimental results. J Neurosurg 75: 1–7

Gugliemi G, Vinuela F, Dion J et al. (1991b) Electrothrombosis of saccular aneurysms via endovascular approach. Part 2: Preliminary clinical experience. J Neurosurg 75: 8–14

Gugleimi G, Vinuela F, Duckweiler G et al. (1992) Endovascular treatment of posterior circulation aneurysms by electrothrombosis using electrically detachable coils. J Neurosurg 77:515–524

Hasan D, Vermeulen M, Wijdicks EFM et al. (1989) Management problems in acute hydrocephalus after subarachnoid haemorrhage. Stroke 20: 747–753

Hodes JE, Aymard A, Gobin YP et al. (1991) Endovascular occlusion of intracranial vessels for curative treatment of unclippable aneurysms: report of 16 cases. J Neurosurg 75: 694–701

Hope AJK, Byrne JV, Molyneux AJ (1999) Factors influencing sucessfull angiographic occlusion of aneurysms treated by coil embolization. American Journal of Neuroradiology 20: 391–399

Higashida RT, Halbach VV, Barnwell SL et al. (1990a) Treatment of Intracranial aneurysms with preservation of the parent vessel: Results of percutaneous balloon embolization in 84 patients. Am J Neuroradiol 11: 633–640

Higashida RT, Halbach VV, Dormandy B et al. (1990b) New microballoon device for transluminal angioplasty of intracranial arterial vasospasm. Am J Neuroradiology 11: 233–238

Hilal SK (1990) Treatment of intracranial aneurysm and arteriovenous malformations with preshaped thrombogenic coils. Am J Neuroradiol 11: 226 (abstract)

Hunt WE, Hess RM (1968) Surgical risks as realted to time of intervention in the repair of intracranial aneurysms. J Neurosurg 28: 14–19

International Study of Unruptured Intracranial Aneurysms (ISUIA) Investigators (1998) Unruptured intracranial aneurysms – risk of rupture and risks of surgical intervention. New England Journal of Medicine 339: 1725–1733

Jane JA, Kassel NF, Torner JC et al. (1985) The natural history of aneurysms and arteriovenous malformations. J Neurosurg 62: 321–323

Jennett B, Bond M (1975) Assessment of outcome after severe brain damage. A practical scale. Lancet i: 480–484

Juvela S, Porras M, Heiskanen O (1993) Natural history of unruptured intracranial aneurysms: a long-term folow-up study. Journal of Neurosurgery 79: 174–182.

Kassel NF, Torner JC, Haley EC et al. (1990a) The international cooperative study on the timing of aneurysm surgery. Part I: overall management results. J Neurosurg 73: 18–36

Kassel NF, Torner JC, Jane JA et al. (1990b) The international cooperative study on the timing of aneurysm surgery. Part II: surgical results. J Neurosurg 73: 37–47

Kassel NF, Helm G, Simmons N et al. (1992) Treatment of cerebral vasospasm with intra-arterial papaverine. J Neurosurg 77: 848–852

Lawton MT, Hamilton MG, Morcoa JJ et al. (1996) Revascularization and aneurysm surgery: Current techniques, indications and outcome. Neurosurgery 38: 83–94

Locksley HB (1966) Report on the Cooperative study of Intracranial Aneurysms and Subarachnoid Haemorrhage: section V. Part II. Natural history of subarachnoid haemorrhage, intracranial aneurysms and arteriovenous malformations. Based on 6268 cases in the cooperative study. J Neurosurg 25: 321–368

Mathis JM, Barr JD, Jungreis CA et al. (1995) Temporary balloon test occlusion of the internal carotid artery: experience in 500 cases. Am J Neuroradiol 16: 749–754

Molyneux AJ, Byrne JV, Renowden S et al. (1996) Endovascular treatment of posterior circulation aneurysms by Guglielmi detachable coils; results in a consecutive series of 100 patients. Neuroradiology 38: 190–194 (Abstract)

Moret J, Cognard C, Weill A et al. (1997) The "remodelling technique" in the treatment of wide neck intracranial aneurysms. Intervent Neuroradiol 3: 21–35

Newell RT, Eskridge JM, Mayberg MR et al. (1989) Angioplasty for treatment of symptomatic vaso spasm following subarachnoid haemorrhage. J Neurosurg 71: 654–660

Peerless SJ, Hernesniemi JA, Gutman FB et al. (1994) Early surgery for ruptured vertebrobasilar aneurysms. J Neurosurg 80: 643–649

Peterman SB, Taylor A Jr, Hoffman JC Jr (1991) Improved detection of cerebral hypoperfusion with internal carotid balloon test occlusion and 99mTc-HMPAO cerebral perfusion SPECT imaging. Am J Neuroradiol 12: 1035–1041

Pierot L, Boulin A, Castaings L (1996) Selective occlusion of basilar artery aneurysms using controlled detachable coils: report of 35 cases. Neurosurgery 38 : 948-954

Rowe JG, Byrne JV, Molyneux A et al. (1996) Endosaccular treatment of intracranial aneurysms. A minimally invasive approach with advantages for elderly patients. Age Ageing 25: 372–376

Rowe JG, Byrne JV, Molyneux A et al. (1995) Haemodynamic consequences of embolizing aneurysms: a transcranial Doppler study. Br J Neurosurg 9: 749–757

-Scotti G, Li MH, Righi C et al. (1996) Endovascular treatment of bactereial intracranial aneurysms. Neuroradiology 38: 186–189

Solomon RA, Fink ME, Pile-Spellman J (1994) Surgical management of unruptured intracranial aneurysms. J Neurosurg 80: 440–446

Serbinenko FA (1974) Balloon catheterization and occlusion of major cerebral vessels. J eurosurg 41: 125–145

Standard SC, Ahuja A, Guterman LR et al. (1995) Balloon test occlusion of the internal carotid artery with hypotensive challenge. Am J Neuroradiol 16: 1453–1458

Steinburg GK, Drake CG, Peerless SJ (1993) Deliberate basilar or vertebral artery occlusion in the treatment of intracranial aneurysms. J Neurosurg 79: 161–173

Sundt TM, Kobayashi S, Fode NC et al. (1982) Results and complications of surgical management of 809 intracranial aneurysms in 722 cases. J Neurosurg 56: 753–765

Tiperman PE, Tomsick TA, Tew JM et al. (1995) Aneurysm formation after carotid occlusion. Am J Neuroradiol 16: 329–331

Van Halbach V, Higashida RT, Dowd CF et al. (1994) The efficacy of endosaccular aneurysm occlusion in alleviating neurological deficits produced by mass effect. J Nueorsurg 80: 659–666

Vinuela F, Duckwiler G, Mawad M (1997) Guglielmi detachable coil embolisation of acute intracranial aneurysms: perioperative anatomical and clinical outcome in 403 patients. J Neurosurg 86: 475–482

Zubillaga AF, Guglielmi G, Vinuela F et al. (1994) Endovascular occlusion of intracranial aneurysms with electrically detachable coils: correlation of aneurysm neck size and treatment results. Am J Neuroradiol 15: 815–820

Chapter 4

Cavernous Sinus Lesions

Robert J. Sellar

Dural Arteriovenous Malformations of the Cavernous Sinus

Classification

Dural arteriovenous malformations (DAVM) or fistulas (DAVF) have traditionally been classified according to their venous drainage (Djindjian 1978 updated by Cognard et al. 1995).

Type I   Drainage into a sinus
Type II Drainage with reflux into cerebral veins
Type III Drainage solely into cortical veins
Type IV Drainage with venous lake.

More recently a simplified classification has been devised by Borden et al. (1995).

Type I   Drainage only into dural sinus or meningeal vein
Type II Drainage into dural sinus and leptomeningeal veins
Type III Drainage into leptomeningeal veins.

The importance of standardising the way in which we classify disease has recently been stressed by Mansmann (1997). It is the only way for different centres to describe comparable groups of patients, thus make valid comparisons of differing treatments, and to identify prognostic factors. To date, only the venous drainage has been definitely identified as a factor influencing natural history. However, the ease of treatment of cavernous carotid fistulas is effected by the rate of flow and type of arterial supply. In 1995 Barrow proposed the following sub-classification (Barrow et al., 1995).

A Fast flowing, typically solitary, communications resulting from traumatic tears of aneurysm rupture.
B Cavernous fistulas supplied only by dural branches of the internal carotid artery.
C Cavernous fistulas supplied only by the dural branches of the external carotid artery.
D Cavernous fistulas supplied by dural branches of both the internal and external carotid artery.

Natural History

On account of the rarity of DAVFs the natural history has been poorly documented. The best attempt has been that of Davies et al. (1997a) who divided their patients into Borden type I (benign) and Borden type II and III (aggressive). Only 2% of type I patients presented with haemorrhage or neurological deficit whereas 39% of grade II and 79% of grade III patients presented with these aggressive symptoms. The outcome of these patients was further documented with 81% of grade I patients improving or being cured without treatment and 86% of those patients treated with embolization. Only one aggressive event was noted in a follow up period totaling 133 patient years (Davies et al., 1997b). This was compared to a haemorrhage rate of 19.2% and mortality of 10.9% per patient year for those with type II or III lesions. It should be noted that local cranial nerve palsies related to cavernous sinus lesions were not considered as a neurological deficit for the purposes of the study.

Aetiology

Dural arteriovenous fistulas frequently occur in association with a venous abnormality. Typically, there is a history indicating an episode of venous thrombosis. Other DAVFs are associated with congenital anomalies of the venous system, including aplasia and stenosis. It is likely that other factors play a part in the development of these lesions as many patients occlude their sinuses without developing a DAVF. There are normal dural arteriovenous connections which may dilate secondary to venous obstruction. It may be that a structural abnormality is also required to develop a DAVM. The vascular tree is a remarkably adaptive structure and depends on a number of factors for remodeling. Gibbons and Dzan (1994) have identified four main factors, cell growth, cell death, cell migration and production or degradation of the extracellular matrix. These processes are set in chain by external factors which may be mechanical, e.g. flow, hormonal or metabolic. The DAVF may be as a result of inappropriate remodelling following a venous injury. These fistulas have been demonstrated antenatally.

Clinical Features (Table 4.1)

The symptoms of DAVMs are secondary to the increased blood flow and the venous intracranial hypertension that results. Patients may complain of a bruit or headaches. Fistulas to the cavernous sinus are the commonest type encountered and may lead to symptoms related to the high pressure in ophthalmic veins and cavernous

Table 4.1. Clinical features of cavernous sinus DAVM

Local	Bruit
	Proptosis
	Visual loss
	Cranial nerve palsies (III, IV, V, VI)
	Glaucoma
	Retinal detachment
General (due to raised intracranial pressure)	Headache
	Papilloedema
	Optic atrophy
Haemorrhage	

sinus include proptosis, visual loss and other cranial nerve palsies. Lesions are described as being high flow or low flow depending on the degree of shunting. High flow lesions are more likely to present with bruits and raised intracranial pressure. In children the flow may be sufficient to cause cardiac failure and hydrocephalus – possibly due to impaired cerebrospinal fluid (CSF) absorption in the presence of high venous sinus pressure.

Symptoms frequently fluctuate and this may be due to on-going thrombosis in the cavernous sinus (Vinuela et al., 1986).

Treatment of Dural AVMs

Treatment options include the following

- Conservative
- Compression of the carotid
- Arterial embolization
- Venous embolization

Conservative Treatment

Conservative treatment is appropriate for elderly, frail patients particularly if the symptoms are mild. A benign venous drainage without cortical reflux is also in favour of an expectant approach. Occasionally, the anatomy of the fistula militates against embolisation, particularly if the malformation is fed by short pedicles arising directly from the internal carotid, and these cases should have a trial of conservative treatment or carotid compression. Surprisingly, a few patients are cured by diagnostic angiography alone, but many more are cured by carotid compression.

Carotid Compression

Carotid compression will cure up to 34% of patients (Van Halbach et al., 1992). Van Halbach recommends compression six times a day for 30 seconds for a period of 4–6 weeks. It is important to stop aspirin, other antiplatelet, or anticoagulation treatment during this period. It is worth demonstrating the technique to the patient. The patient should use the opposite hand to compress their carotid so that if cerebral ischaemia occurs the manual pressure stops. The patient should be sitting in case of a vasovagal attack. In order to induce thrombosis the carotid and venous flows should both be compressed and any bruit should disappear. This treatment is not recommended for patients with cortical venous drainage.

Arterial Embolisation

Until recently, this was the preferred option for treating DAVMs. The cure rate using this approach is 70–80%. Picard et al., (1987) reported on using particle embolisation in 25 cases of DAVFs with a cure rate of 72% and improvement in 24%. He had one death due to particles penetrating an anastomosis between the internal and external carotid artery. Vinuela also reported a case of hemiparesis following glue embolization (Vinuela et al., 1984). Van Halbach reported a series of 45 patients–78% of patients were cured; there were four patients who suffered permanent complications (Van Halbach et al., 1992). Complications included Vth nerve hyperaesthesia following glue embolisation of the accessory, meningeal and visual loss following particles entering the meningolacrimal branch of the middle meningeal artery. Glue has the advantage of penetrating the fistula but also may enter unseen anastamoses (Figure 4.1). Particles need to be 150 μm to avoid embolisation of arteries to the cranial nerves given of by meningeal vessels but if they are too big occlusion proximal to the fistula and allows for recruitment of collaterals. It

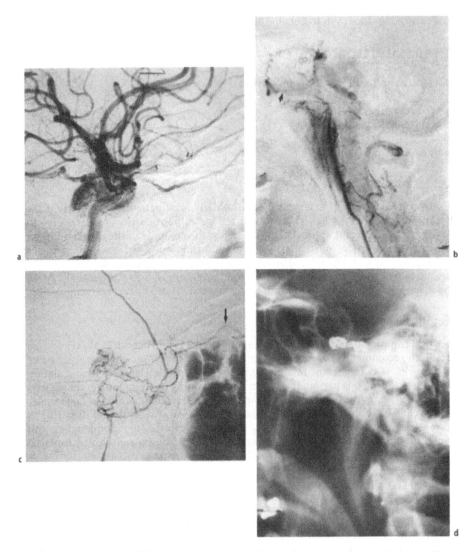

Fig. 4.1. Cavernous sinus dural fistula. **a** Left internal carotid injection; reveals shunting into the posterior cavernous sinus. The fistula is not well seen. **b** Right ascending pharyngeal artery injection. The pharyngeal trunk anastomoses with the maxillary artery via the pterygovaginal artery (small arrow) and then to the fistula via the artery of the foramen rotundum. Note the filling of the vertebral artery. **c** Left selective middle meningeal injection. This reveals multiple small feeders to the fistula. Unfortunately, there is a large meningo lacrinal branch (large arrow) compare this with the distal artery with the ophthalmic artery seen on the internal carotid injection. Such anastomoses are a contraindication to using arterial emboli particularly glue. **d** The fistula was successfully treated using a transvenous approach with fibre coils.

is very important to be aware of potential connections between the external carotid and the internal carotid or the vertebral arteries; these may open up during embolisation and repeated control angiograms should be performed if the catheter position is proximal to any known potential connection. Embolisation of branches of the internal carotid artery is only rarely performed since reflux has the potential to cause dire consequences, but if all other treatment fails and the microcatheter can be satisfactorily wedged in either the meningohypophyseal or inferolateral trunk then careful embolisation is possible. A non-detachable balloon can be used to protect the carotid if particles are being used.

Transvenous

The transvenous approach has become the treatment of choice for most DAVFs. The inferior petrosal vein is approached via the jugular vein. Catheterisation may prove difficult on account of the multiple valves faced when travelling from the femoral vein. A terumo guide wire is useful for gently probing the valves. The most common obstruction is at the site of entry of the internal jugular vein into the subclavian vein. A catheter with a simple curve such as head hunter is usually sufficient for negotiating the venous pathway. As the jugular bulb can be exquisitely sensitive to internal pressure, we use a microcatheter to find the inferior petrosal sinus. It is often difficult to be precise about the site of the fistulae into the cavernous sinus. A useful classification of fistulas of the cavernous sinus has recently been given by Usami et al. (1998); they draw a line dividing the cavernous sinus in half (this line divides the cavernous carotid artery into two equal parts) fistulas that enter the sinus above the line are considered more dangerous to treat as the superior ophthalmic vein may be occluded and since most of the cortical veins to the cavernous sinus enter into this area venous hypertension is most likely to occur if this area is packed.

Van Halbach reported 54 patients of whom 81% were cured by a transvenous approach and has adopted this as the treatment of choice (Van Halbach et al., 1987).

Treatment Aims and Choices

Treatment choice depends on severity of symptoms and anatomical classification. Those with mild symptoms are given a trial of conservative treatment with carotid compression for 6 weeks. Patients who have more serious symptoms can be treated initially trans arterially particularly if all the feeders are from the external carotid but most cases are now approached trans venously after obliterating the main arterial feeders. If the inferior petrosal sinus is thrombosed the fistula can be approached directly via the superior ophthalmic vein or by the angular vein (Teng et al., 1995).

Carotid Cavernous Fistula

Introduction

Endovascular treatment of carotid cavernous fistulas (CCF) with detachable balloons is one of the few new medical treatments that was seen immediately to be so superior to previously available surgical methods of treatment that comparative trials have not been necessary. Exploration of the cavernous sinus presents many practical problems for surgeons and usually entails temporary clamping of the internal carotid but occlusion of the fistula by endovascular techniques provides a solution that is elegant, simple and nearly always successful (Vinuela et al., 1984; Debrun et al., 1988).

Aetiology

The most frequent cause of a CCF is following trauma; often there is an associated facial fracture. The tear typically occurs at the two points of fixation of the carotid – by its dural attachment as it exits the carotid canal and the more distal dural attachment just below the anterior clinoid process.

Carotid aneurysms may rupture into the cavernous sinus resulting in a fistula. This usually occurs in older patients. Finally, there are occasional reports of iatrogenic CCFs caused by attempted treatment through the foramen ovale for trigeminal neuralgia (Guglielmi et al., 1995) and thrombectomy for carotid atheroma (Debrun, 1992).

Traumatic CCFs may be bilateral and occasionally two tears in one carotid have been found.

Pathophysiology

The fistula is typically 2–5 mm in diameter. A high flow fistula nearly always develop on account of the pressure difference between the arterial and venous circulations. The cavernous sinus dilates and retrograde flow occurs most frequently into the superior and inferior ophthalmic veins but also across the midline to the other cavernous sinus. A more worrying sign is when reflux is seen into cortical veins, when there is a real risk of intracerebral haemorrhage.

Clinical Features

Surprisingly, the clinical features do not appear immediately but usually after several days and sometimes not for several weeks. The patient often then becomes aware of a bruit. Proptosis of the globe with chemosis are then the next commonest presenting features. This may be followed by palsies of the cranial nerves that traverse the walls of the cavernous sinus (III, IV, V and VI). Pain may be experienced along the distribution of the Vth nerve.

Treatment is required urgently if hemiparesis develops secondary to venous hypertension or if the ocular pressure exceeds 40 mmHg. A rare complications is epistaxis, which can be torrential if there is erosion through the thin-walled sphenoid sinus (Gelbert et al., 1986; Kuipersmith et al., 1986).

The long-term outlook for an untreated CC fistula is poor with some 50% of patients going on to lose their vision on the affected site (Kuipersmith et al., 1986).

Treatment

Surgical treatment by carotid ligation is not usually successful as direct exposure of the fistula is a complex operation. Stereotactic radiotherapy can be used for low flow situations, but this is seldom seen in direct CCfs (Barcia-Salorio). Small holes are typically caused by iatrogenically and these can be treated by GDC coils (Guglielmi et al., 1995; Siniluoto Seppanen et al., 1997).

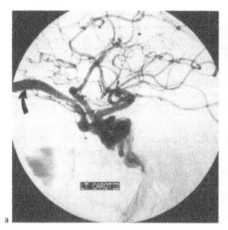 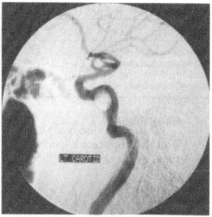

Fig. 4.2 **a** Internal carotid angiogram reveals a high-flow carotid cavernous fistula with reflux into the superior ophthalmic vein (arrow). This resulted in severe left chemosis and proptosis. **b** Treatment with a detachable silicone balloon: the microcatheter at this stage is still attached and shows the site of fistula in the precavernous carotid – a common site for traumatic fistula.

Balloon embolisation of the CCF is the mainstay of treatment. This was first performed by Serbinenko (1974) but the technique was popularized by Debrun using latex balloons attached to a microcatheter with latex string (Debrun et al., 1988). More recently balloons have been developed with valves that allow the balloon to be placed and then detached with gentle pressure – either from a coaxial catheter which is passed up to the balloon or more commonly by inflating the balloon in the cavernous sinus and then gently pulling the microcatheter off the balloon. Silicone balloons are made with a detachable valve mechanism and are easier to use. Silicone is semipermeable and, therefore, needs to be filled with isotonic contrast medium. The force required to detach the ballon has been graded high, medium or low. We use medium, detachable, silicone balloons (DSB) routinely (Figure 4.2). On one occasion during the treatment of a very high flow CCF, a balloon has prematurely detached but the flow sucked the balloon into a safe position in the cavernous sinus.

Technique

Angiographic Assessment

Full angiographic assessment is as shown in Table 4.2. Lateral series are the most valuable although an anteroposterior series of the ipsilateral carotid artery is performed to show reflux into cortical veins and across the cavernous sinus. Cross-compression studies are used if occlusion of the carotid is contemplated and also may help to show the level of fistula. A vertebral injection also may help to identify the level of the fistula.

Anaesthesia

It is preferable to perform this procedure under general anaesthesia (GA) as balloon inflation may stretch the dura of the cavernous sinus and the associated nerves

Table 4.2. Angiographic assessment of CCF

Vessel	Purpose
Ipsilateral internal carotid artery	To establish diagnosis
Ipsilateral vertebral artery	Will often establish level of CCF
Contralateral internal carotid artery	Excludes bilateral CCF, occlusion or aneurysm
Bilateral external carotid arteries	Less important: occasional fistulous connection

leading to pain. GA does not allow testing for occulomotor palsy or for cerebral perfusion if complete occlusion of the carotid is required, this should only be performed after awake test occlusion.

Treatment

Arterial Approach
The arterial approach is successful in 80–90% of the cases (Higashida et al., 1989., Lewis et al., 1995). A balloon is selected on an estimate of the size of the fistula and the degree of dilation of the cavernous sinus. The hole in the carotid is often not directly visualized but inferred by the rate of flow volume of the contrast entering the cavernous sinus. Balloons are now available in many different sizes and shapes, the typical range used vary from 4 mm up to 22 mm when dilated. Debrun uses latex balloons and usually starts with medium sized balloons that are 7–10 mm diameter when inflated. If the balloon fails to cross through to the cavernous sinus spontaneously, the balloon can be slightly inflated and the flow may then suck it through. Steaming a curve on the microcatheter may also assist the transit of the balloon through the fistula. Finally, changing the balloon to a small diameter balloon may be necessary if the fistula is small. Occasionally, complete occlusion is not obtained with a single balloon and multiple balloons are necessary. A small residual leak will often spontaneously heal (check angiography at 1 week is recommended). If the symptoms persist and the balloon is preventing the placement of a more suitably sized balloon then it is possible to puncture via the foramen ovale (Jacobs et al., 1993). If this approach fails a venous approach is attempted.

Venous Sinus Approach
The cavernous sinus can be catheterized via the jugular vein and inferior petrosal sinus. This is most easily accomplished using a wire directed microcatheter, e.g. a Tracker 10 or 18 or Prowler catheters (Boston Scientific, Cordis). Through the microcatheter coils can be deposited in the cavernous sinus opposite the fistula. If the cavernous sinus is over-packed, particularly anteriorly, there is a small risk of obstructing the orbital veins with subsequently thrombosis (Vinuela et al., 1984). This may lead to a transient deterioration in symptoms and rarely blindness. The new vortex GDC coils with attached fibres (Boston Scientific) are particularly suitable for inducing thrombosis.

Ophthalmic Vein Approach
Several authors have reported success using either direct puncture or surgical exposure of the ophthalmic veins (Teng et al., 1995). Direct puncture at the superior orbital fissure may result in temporary ptosis.

If none of these methods succeed carotid arterial occlusion will usually cure the fistula. Placement of the balloon across the fistula can be problematical if the fistula is close to the ophthalmic artery and this also occluded by the balloon (but surgical clipping of the ophthalmic artery only results in blindness in 10% of patients and has seldom been recorded secondary to balloon occlusion). If the balloon cannot be placed across the fistula then balloons above and below the fistula can be deployed.

Whichever method of occlusion, check angiography should be performed at 6 months to exclude a pseudo-arterial aneurysm and to confirm complete cure of the fistula.

Results

The results of two large series are remarkably consistent with a 90% success rate via the arterial route and the remainder via the venous route (Higashida et al., 1989; Lewis, et al., 1995).

Common complications are those of cranial nerve palsy but these often resolve over several months. Lewis et al. reported a 4% complication rate including cerebral infarction and one death in their 100 cases. This related to a balloon that moved and resulted in major cerebral infarction.

Cavernous Aneurysms and Paraclinoid Aneurysms

Aneurysms of the cavernous sinus need to be carefully classified if they are to be correctly managed. Aneurysms may either arise from within the cavernous sinus, expand out of it or, conversely, arise above the dural ring and project back into the cavernous sinus.

Classification

Cavernous Aneurysms

- Anterio genu
- Horizontal segment
- Posterior genu

Cavernous aneurysms commonly arise from the horizontal segment or the anterior genu of the carotid. The importance of the distinction is that aneurysms of the anterior genu may point into the chiasmatic cisterns and produce subarachnoid haemorrhage.

Paraclinoid Aneurysms

These have been subdivided by Ogilvy (1995) into five groups; three of these groups of aneurysms lie above the cavernous sinus and therefore are beyond the remit of this chapter (aneurysms that arise at the ophthalmic artery origin which often project upwards, posterior carotid wall aneurysms which typically project posterolaterally and most distally the superior hypophyseal aneurysm which projects upwards and medially frequently compressing the optic nerve). The most proximal aneurysms are, however, relevant. These are the transitional aneurysms which starts from within the cavernous sinus and projects upwards through the dural ring towards the chiasmatic cistern and the carotid cave aneurysm which has its neck above the ring but projects inferiorly to the clinoid process into the cavernous sinus. Clearly, both of these aneurysms, which partly lie below and partly above the clinoid dural rings, may present with subarachnoid haemorrhage.

Clinical Presentation

Carotid aneurysms are commonly asymptomatic. When they expand they often compress the cranial nerves that run in and along the wall of the cavernous sinus. The commonest nerve to be compressed in VI followed by III and IV. This leads to diploplia and ptosis. The fifth nerve, when compressed, gives rise to facial numbness or facial pain – this may be exquisite, disrupting sleep and making the patient feel suicidal.

Rarer presentations include those of massive epitaxis if the sphenoid sinus is eroded. The medial wall of the cavernous sinus rarely may be breached with reluctant subarachnoid haemorrhage. Finally, emboli from the aneurysm sac can lead to ischaemic episodes or a stroke presentation.

Treatment of Cavernous Aneurysms

Indications

Cavernous aneurysms are often found in elderly patients who are asymptomatic. There is little justification in treating these patients. Some authors draw a distinction between those aneurysms that are likely to cause subarachnoid haemorrhage and those that only rarely do so. These authors recommend treatment of anterior genu aneurysms which frequently point medially into the subarachnoid space, these same authors believe that MRI can reliably detect the direction of the aneurysm (Linskey et al., 1990).

Other indications for treatment of asymptomatic aneurysms are those that have eroded into the sinuses, giant aneurysms and paraclinoid aneurysms all of which are prone to complications. It should be stressed that there is little evidence for these recommendations and final decisions are often heavily influenced by the age, fitness, and attitudes of the patient.

The commonest indication of treatment is the development of opthalmoplegia or facial pain. The natural history is typically progressive once symptoms start and if the patient is in good health early treatment is recommended (Ogilvy, 1995).

Treatment Options

Cavernous aneurysms can be treated surgically, but on account of the technical difficulties of opening the cavernous sinus most cavernous aneurysms are now treated using interventional techniques. Three techniques are commonly used: balloon occlusion of the parent vessel, coiling with GDC and coiling in association with a remodelling balloon. The decision of which technique to use depends on the age of the patient, toleration of temporary occlusion of the carotid and the width of the aneurysm neck.

Balloon Occlusion
Many cavernous carotid aneurysms are wide necked and unsuitable for coiling. Balloon occlusion of the carotid parent artery is then the treatment of choice. Test occlusion of the carotid artery is performed first.

Test Occlusion There is considerable variability in the technique used. Our own view is that many of the tests such as xenon CT scanning after temporary occlusion make the procedure more complicated and probably add to the risks by having to move the patient without predicting with any reliability which patients will tolerate balloon occlusion. Although such techniques have enthusiastic proponents no statistical evidence has ever been produced to show that they confer any advantage (Little et al., 1989; Yonas et al., 1992). We keep to a simple protocol. The patient is antiocaogulated with heparin (5–10 000 units). Angiography with cross compression is performed to demonstrate reasonable flow across the circle of Willis. Then the carotid artery is occluded with a silicone detachable balloon and the patient is monitored carefully over 20 minutes for any symptoms or signs of ischaemia. If there are none the balloon is detached.

There are two modifications that should be mentioned. These do not involve moving the patient and possibly improve the safety of the procedure. First, a balloon mounted on a double lumen catheter can be used. This allows the distal stump pressure to be measured. Pressures below 50 mmHg systolic indicate a high probability of secondary ischaemia. Jawad concluded that stump pressures of 60 mmHg or over are desirable (Jawad et al., 1977). Second, it is relatively straightforward to challenge the cerebral perfusion reserve by reducing the blood pressure 20–30 mmHg. This is a straightforward procedure that the anaesthetists can achieve simply with an antihypertensive such as hydralazine. Recently, the New York group have reduced their complication rate by first assessing the patency of the circle of Willis and the collateral circulation from the external carotid arteries (Niima et al., 1996). Patients with "poor" collateral circulation do not undergo test occlusion (unfortunately "poor" is not defined). By using a double lumen balloon catheter they are able to measure stump pressure. Surprisingly, they have ended up not using this measurement believing that it is a poor predictor of stroke risk. Instead they inject contrast to assess the rate of washout due to collateral flow. The literature is full of such idiosyncratic approaches to test occlusion. However, using this technique they reduced their risks of permanent occlusion from 16 to 0% for their last 47 cases. The crucial change in their protocol was probably the introduction of stringent post occlusion care; maintaining the blood pressure and PO_2.

Patients who have unsuitable anatomy or who fail test occlusion should be considered for EC-IC bypass or for one of the other techniques, e.g. coil embolisation (s/b) which preserve the parent vessel.

Balloon Occlusion (Permanent) We do not see any clear-cut advantage in measuring stump pressures, wash out rates or performing any of the blood flow tests that can be undertaken during test occlusion. The same balloon is used, therefore, the same balloon that is detached to make a permanent occlusion (ITC silicone balloon). Silicone balloons are softer than latex. They have been designed with self sealing valves which prevent deflation after the microcatheter has been withdrawn. The valves are available requiring three different levels of detachment traction. For most purposes, the medium valve is suitable. It is important though to inflate the balloon through the microcatheter using isotonic contrast as silicone is semipermeable.

There is considerable debate as to whether aneurysms should be isolated from the circulation by placing balloons above and below the neck (Niima et al., 1996). Most centres do not feel that this is necessary and that it has the disadvantage of sometimes sacrificing the ophthalmic artery. There is also the theoretical risk of aneurysm rupture, since the distal balloon is typically inflated first. The preferred method is to occlude the carotid either at the neck of the aneurysm or just below the

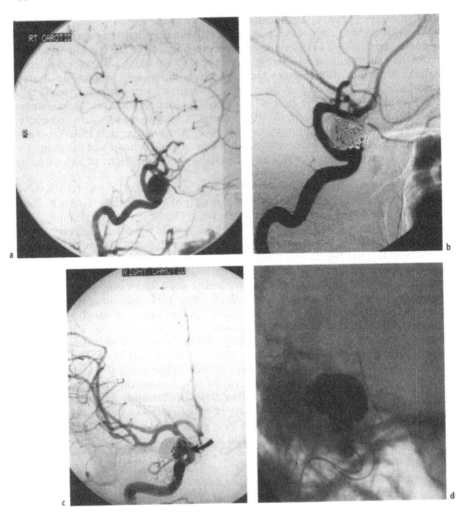

Fig. 4.3. Paraclinoid aneurysm. **a** Common carotid artery injection. There is a large, broad-necked aneurysm arising close to the origin of the ophthalmic artery. **b** Coiling of the aneurysm. **c** Three months post procedure check angiography reveals coil compaction. **d** Recoiling of the aneurysm neck using the "remodelling" technique; note the inflated balloon which allows much tighter packing of the coils. **e** After balloon deflation the coils can be seen to be flattened to form part of the internal carotid wall. Check angiography at 6 months confirmed no regrowth of the aneurysm (opposite page).

neck. This is followed up by a second more proximal balloon. A solid clot rapidly forms between the two balloons reducing the chance of late balloon migration (Figure 4.4). Typically, the aneurysm will then shrink or clot on follow-up MRI. If there is collateral circulation via the external carotid artery a sump balloon placed at the origin of the internal carotid artery may reduce emboli from this source.

Post-operative Care

It is the 48 hours after the balloon occlusion that is critical in preventing stroke. It is important to monitor blood pressure and also ensure that the patient does not

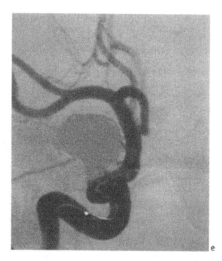

Fig. 4.3. e

become hypoxic. For this purpose our patients are observed in a high dependency unit. A particularly high risk time is during transfer from the angiography suite back to the ward. We have found hypotension frequently occurring in transit. The patient should be nursed flat for the first 48 hours and then gradually have their head elevated during this time. With close attention to postoperative care, we have had one transient complication occurring 4 weeks post procedure (32 patients).

Other Treatments: Coiling and Remodelling

Coiling of cavernous aneurysms is a feasible alternative, particularly if the aneurysms is small. Unfortunately, cavernous aneurysms frequently are greater than 1.5 cm in diameter and may have considerable intraluminal clot. Coils in such aneurysms both compact and migrate into the clot (Figure 4.3), successful long-term exclusion of the aneurysm being achieved in only 50% of cases.

Frequently, these aneurysms have wide necks and coiling them carries considerable risk of coil prolapse into the parent artery. These wide necked aneurysms can be treated by the remodelling technique popularized by Moret et al., (1997). This involves inflating a pliable, small balloon (3 mm diameter and 1 cm in length) across the aneurysm neck whilst coils are being introduced. Aneurysms can then be firmly packed without fear of prolapse of coils into the parent artery. After deflation the coils maintain their modelled shape (Fig 4.3e). This technique should be done with higher doses of heparin to achieve activated clotting time (ACT) levels of 4-5, as well as aspirin to reduce platelet aggregation.

Conclusion

There are several interventional approaches for treating cavernous aneurysms including parent vessel occlusion, coiling and coiling without remodelling. The treatment of choice depends on careful analysis of the morphology of the aneurysm and the functional status of the rest of the cerebral circulation and the fitness of the individual patient.

References

Barcia-Salorio JL, Soler F, Barcia JA et al. Radiosurgery of carotid cavernous fistulae.
Barrow DC, Spector RH, Braun IF, Candman JA, Tindall SC, Tindall GT (1985) Classification and treatment of carotid cavernous sinus fistulas. J Neurosurg 62: 248–256
Borden JA, Wu JK, Shucart WA (1995) A proposed classification for spinal and cranial dural arteriovenous fistulous malformations and implications for treatment. J Neurosurg 82: 166–179
Cognard C, Gobin YP et al. (1995) Cerebral dural arteriovenous fistulas: clinical and angiographic correlation with a revised classification of venous drainage. Radiology 194: 671–680
Davies M, Saleh J, Ter Brugge K, Willinski R, Wallace MC (1997a) The natural history and management of intracranial dural arteriovenous fistulae. Part 1: benign lesions. Intervent Neuradio 3: 295–302
Davies MA, Ter Brugge K, Willinski, Wallace M (1997b) The natural history and management of intracranial dural arteriovenous fistulae. Part II: aggressive lesions. Intervent Neuroradio 3: 303–311
Debrun GM, Vinuela F, Fox AJ, Davis KR, Ahn, HS (1988) Indications for treatment and classification of 132 CCFs. Neurosurgery 22: 285–289
Debrun G (1992) Management of traumatic carotid cavernous fistulas. In: Interventional neuroradiology: endovascular therapy of the central nervous system. Raven Press, New York, p 107
Gelbert F, Reizine D, Stecken I, Ruffenacht D, Laffont J, Merland JJ (1986) Severe epitasis by rupture of the ICA into the sphenoid sinus. J Neuroradio 13: 163–171
Gibbons GH, Dzau VJ (1994) The emerging concept of vascular remodelling. N Engl J Med 20: 1432–1438
Guglielmi G, Vinueza F, Duckwiler G, Dion J Stocker A (1995) High flow small hole arteriovenous fistulas treatment with electrodetachable coils. AJNR 16: 325–328
Higashida RT, Halbach VV, Tsai FD et al. (1989) Interventional neurovascular treatment of traumatic carotid and vertebral artery lesions. Results in 234 cases. AJR 153: 577–582
Inmat F, Ferrer E, Twose J (1986) Direct intracavernous obliteration of high flow CCF. J Neurosurg 65: 770–775
Jacobs JM, Parker GD, Apfelbaum RI (1993) Deflation of detachable balloons in the cavernous sinus by percutaneous puncture. AJNR 14: 175–177
Jawad K, Miller JD, Wyper DJ et al. (1977) Measurement of CBF and carotid artery pressure compared with cerebral angiography in assessing collateral blood supply after carotid ligation. J Neurosurg 46: 185–186
Kupiersmith M, Berenstein A, Flamm E et al. (1986) Neuro-ophthamologic abnormalities and intravascular therapy of traumatic carotid cavernous fistulas. Ophthalmology 93: 906–912
Lewis AI, Tomsick TA, Tew JM Jr (1995) Management of 100 consecutive direct carotid–cavernous fistulas: results of treatment with detachable balloon. Neurosurgery 36: 239–244
Linskey ME, Sekhar CN, Hirsh WC et al. (1990) Aneurysms of the internal carotid artery; natural history and indications for treatment. Neurosurgery 26: 933–938
Little JR, Rosenfeld JV, Awad IA (1989) Internal carotid artery occlusion for cavernous segment aneurysm. Neurosurgery 25: 398–404
Mansmann U (1997) Making evidence available prognostic classification systems. Intervent Neuroradio 3: 289–293
Moret J, Cognard et al. (1997) The "remodelling technique" in the treatment of wide neck intracranial aneurysms. Angiographic results and clinical FU in 56 cases. Intervent Neuroradio 3: 21–35
Niima Y, Berenstein A, Setton A, Kupersmith MJ (1996) Occlusion of the internal carotid artery based on a simple tolerance test. Int Neuroradio 2: 289–296
Ogilvy CS (1995) Paraclinoid carotid aneurysms. In Ojemann A, Ogilvy CS, Crowell RM, Heros RC (eds) Surgical management of neurovascular disease, 3rd edn. Williams and Wilkin, Baltimore, pp 185–213
Picard C, Bracard S, Maccet J, Per A, Glacobbe HC, Roland J (1987) Spontaneous dural arteriovenous fistulas. Semin Intervent Radiol 4: 219–240
Siniluoto Seppanen T, Seppanew S, Kuurne T, Wilkholm G, Leinonen S, Svenosen P (1997) Transarterial embolisation of a direct carotid cavernous fistula with detachable coils. AJNR 18: 519–523
Teng MM, Lirng JF, Chang T et al. (1995) Embolisation of carotid cavernous fistula by means of direct puncture through the superior orbital fissure. Radiology 194: 705–711
Serbinenko FA (1974) Balloon catheterization and occlusion of major cerebral vessels. J Neurosurg 41: 125–145

Usami S, Abet, Hatay (1998) Embolisation method for cavernous sinus fistula within the cavernous sinus. Int Neuroradio 4: 213–218

Halbach VV, Hiesema GB, Higashida RT, Reicher M (1987) Carotid cavernous fistula: indications for urgent treatment. AJNR 8: 627–633

Halbach VV, Higashida RI, Hieshema GB, Dowd CF (1992) Endovascular therapy of dural fistulas in: Vineula (ed) Interventional neuroradiology. Raven Press ltd, New York, pp 29–50

Vinuela F, Fox AT, Debrun GM, Peerless SJ, Drake CG (1984) Spontaneous carotid–cavernous fistulas clinical, radiological and therapeutic considerations. Experience in 20 cases. J Neurosurg 60(s): 976–984

Vinuela FV, Fox AJ et al. (1986) Unusual clinical manifestations of dural arteriovenous malformations. J Neurosurg 64: 554–558

Yonas H, Linskey M et al. (1992) Internal carotid balloon test occlusion does require quantitative CBF. Am J Neuroradio 13: 1147–1148

Chapter 5

Cerebral Arteriovenous Malformations

Robert J. Sellar

Introduction

The patient with a cerebral arteriovenous malformation (AVM) poses the clinician with some of the hardest management choices in medicine. No two patients with AVMs have the same prognosis and it requires considerable medical knowledge of risk factors and angioarchitecture to evolve the correct management strategy for an individual patient.

There are several reasons why such management decisions are difficult. First, there is no consensus as to how AVMs should be classified or even defined. Surgical classifications do not concur with radiological classifications since different anatomical factors lead to morbidity from the interventional radiological and surgical treatment (Spetzler & Martin, 1986). Recently, the results of radiosurgery have been shown to be largely independent of the factors that make up the Spetzler-Martin Grading (Meder et al.). The distinction between a nidal AVM as opposed to a fistula has never been clearly made. These definitions require clarification as radiosurgery has poor results where there is a high-flow fistula, whereas embolisation is often successful in this situation.

Second, AVMs are rare, with an incidence of approximately one-tenth of that of cerebral aneurysms. There are 10–15 new cases per million population per year. Although some pathological series, such as that of Jellinger (1986), have found an autopsy incidence as high as 0.14% but his group includes patients with venous anomalies (Figure 5.1) and telangectasias. This has meant that even reports from large centres have small numbers of patients and that no treatment has yet been put through the "acid test" of a randomised, controlled trial.

Third, the natural history of AVMs is imperfectly known. Most authors compare their results of treatment with historical series but these historical series comprise highly selected groups of patients often taken from larger groups that have been treated.

Finally, there are three disciplines, surgery, radiology and radiotherapy, all offering their own treatments and each with proponents that are prepared to suggest an occasion that treatments other than their own chosen method are tantamount to being unethical (Heros, 1997). Unfortunately, there have not been very randomised trials for any of the treatments of AVMs to back up their assertions.

This chapter will attempt to look critically at the evidence that is available to help the clinician decide how to manage their individual patient.

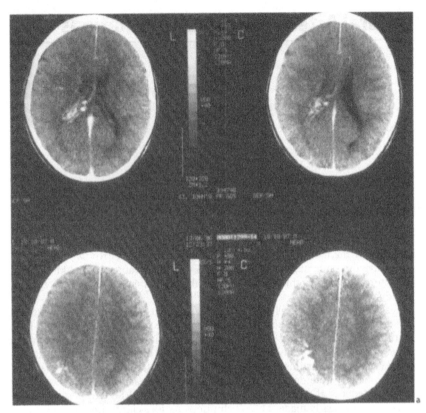
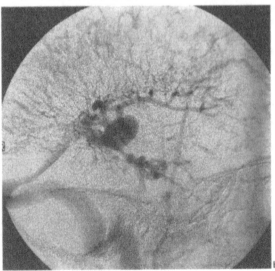

Fig. 5.1. Venous anomaly in a 13-year-old boy with Von recklinghausen disease. **a** CT scan suggestive of an arteriovenous malformation. **b** Venous phase DSA demonstrating this to be a venous anomaly; risk of haemorrhage nil, intervention dangerous.

Classification of Brain AVMs

The first step towards successful management of a brain AVM is to correctly classify the lesion. This should be a four-stage procedure. The first two stages are a morphological classification of AVMs and this is usually straightforward.

Morphological Classification (after McCormick (1962))

- Cerebral arteriovenous malformations
- Cavernous haemangiomas
- Telangectasias
- Venous anomalies (Figure 5.1).

Only cerebral arteriovenous malformations, of this broad classification, will be considered in this chapter.

- Single
- Multiple
    Familial
    Non-familial

Multiple AVMs

Multiple cerebral arteriovenous malformations may be sporadic or familial. In the experience of Willinski et al. (1990), about 25% were part of the Osler-Weber-Rendu syndrome. These patients have multiple telangectasias of the gastrointestinal (GI) tract as well as lung and brain arteriovenous malformations. Patients may, therefore, present with a brain abscess secondary to emboli from an infected lung AV fistula rather than a bleed. The Wyburn-Mason syndrome consists of cutaneous naevi and cerebral AVMs. Theron et al. (1974) found there was common involvement of the optic nerve and visual pathways (22 out of 25 patients).

The risk of brain haemorrhage and other sequalae from these familial and multiple AVMs is not well documented and is assumed to be the same as for AVMs occurring in isolation. Osler-Weber-Rendu malformations frequently have anomalous venous drainage and this should be carefully assessed prior to treatment (Figure 5.1) which is seldom indicated as these are venous anomalies.

Surgical Classification

The early grading systems used by neurosurgeons lacked any consistency, especially regarding diameter. Many systems classified AVMs under 2 cm as small other defined small AVMs as those under 3 cm. These systems have been reviewed by Martin and Spetzler and recently, the Spetzler-Martin scale has become generally accepted as the most useful surgical classification (Table 5.1). The authors have prospectively evaluated their scale and shown that it can be used to predict surgical morbidity.

Endovascular Classification

This depends heavily on the angioarchitecture of the AVM. Several classifications have been produced (Yasargil, 1987; Haoudart et al., 1993). The simple classification

Table 5.1. Spetzler–Martin classification of AVMs

Graded feature	Points assigned
Size of AVM	
Small (<3 cm)	1
Medium (3–6 cm)	2
Large (>6 cm)	3
Eloquence of adjacent brain	
Non-eloquent	0
Eloquent	1
Pattern of venous drainage	
Superficial only	0
Deep	1

used in Edinburgh below takes into account only the features of an AVM that are important for interventional treatment.

Arterial

- Number of feeding arteries and Site
- Transit or terminal arteries feeding AVM nidus
- Meningeal arteries present or absent
- Flow aneurysms
- Arterial stenoses

Nidus

- Size
- Diffuse architecture
- Gyral involvement rather than sulcal site of AVM
- Perinidal angiogenesis
- Number of compartments
- Fistula (present or absent)
- Aneurysm (present or absent).

Venous

- Number of draining veins
- Venous stenoses
- Varices.

The angioarchitecture has a bearing on four factors.

1. Risk of haemorrhage
2. Risk of embolisation
3. Likelihood of obliteration
4. Likelihood of relieving symptoms.

The risk of haemorrhage is increased with the following factors:

- Clinical factors
    Age over 60
    Recent haemorrhage

- Angiographic Factors
  Flow aneurysm
  Nidal aneurysm
  Nidal fistulae
  Single venous outflow
  Venous stenoses.

Factors that increase the risk of embolisation are as follows:

- Distal AVM; unable to reach nidus for embolisation
- Large (> 6 cm) diameter
- Fed by perforators or small feeders
- Transit vessels that supply a gyral AVM and also normal brain
- Flow aneurysm
- Single draining vein
- Eloquent area.

The decision to treat an individual patient with an AVM requires balancing the natural history of the disease and in particular the risk of haemorrhage against the risk of embolization.

Natural History

Problems with Natural History Studies

The golden age of natural history studies has now passed, since few patients now escape without their AVMs being interfered with by some manner of therapy. Unfortunately, the studies that do exist on groups of untreated patients present many problems of interpretation. There is the inherent bias in most studies in that the patients studied have typically already presented with haemorrhage or seizures. This immediately selects a group in whom the haemodynamic balance has become unstable. None of the small group of patients in Crawford's series who had incidental asymptomatic AVMs, bled during 20 years follow up. (Crawford et al., 1986).

Most of the other series reporting the natural history suffer from other selection bias. (Graf et al., 1983; Fults & Kelly, 1984; Brown et al., 1988, Ondra et al., 1990) Those patients who remain untreated typically include a far greater number of patients who have large AVMs in surgically inaccessible sites. These studies were also performed before the era of superselective angiography and, therefore, the analysis of the AVM anatomy is often inaccurate. For example, recent analysis of angioarchitecture has revealed many AVMs to be smaller than previously thought especially when collateral arteries and draining veins are excluded from the nidal diameter. Likewise, the incidence of associated aneurysms previously thought to be in the region of 8–10% may be as high as 50% if superselective angiography is performed (Turjman et al., 1994). Patients who have fatal bleeds from AVMs also fail to enter into these series, therefore the mortality figures quoted below need to be adjusted by 10–30% to take this into account (Pollock et al., 1996). Finally, all the studies have small groups of patients, only Crawford's series followed more than 200 patients (Crawford et al., 1986). The reader should approach the literature with these caveats in mind.

Overall Morbidity and Mortality

The study that is least effected by bias was initially reported by Troupp et al. in 1965 which was subsequently updated by Ondra et al. (1990). The patients were studied prospectively, all patients were symptomatic, and none had been surgically treated. This was a population-based study including approximately 90% of the Finnish population. One hundred and sixty patients were evaluated for a mean period of 23.7 years. The overall mortality was 1% per year with a severe morbidity of 2.7% per year. The annual rebleed rate was 4%. Two results were surprising, first, the yearly mortality and major morbidity remained constant throughout the follow up period and, second, the mode of presentation did not affect either of these outcomes.

The largest single center study is that done by Crawford et al. (1986) with 345 patients. This study illustrates well the problems of most of the available natural history studies. It is retrospective, follow-up is incomplete with only 76% patients found at publication. It is likely that many patients that were not found had poor outcome. Of the 217 patients that were followed up as the "unoperated group" 13 were subsequently operated on. Of those that died, 37 patients, nine (24%) died at presentation. These deaths are problematic as they are irrelevant when advising a patient who has come as far as requiring counselling in the clinic. On the other hand, if the true overall mortality is required, then deaths of all those who died before admission should be included. Surprisingly, a high proportion of the deaths were not related to haemorrhage (24/26) 52%. The overall results, with an average of 10.4 years follow-up of their patients using life survival analysis, were that there was a 20-year risk of death of 29% and a 42% risk of recurred haemorrhage. The annual risk of death from an AVM calculated from these two disparate sources is remarkably similar.

These series, including the other smaller series of Anderson et al. (1988), Fults & Kelly (1984), Graf et al. (1983) and Brown et al. (1988) have been reviewed by Wilkins (1990); he concludes, with Samson and Barter, that the overall haemorrhage rate for cerebral AVMs is 3–4% per year and that the risk of death from each haemorrhage is 10–15% and that the annual mortality rate is 1% with a risk of permanent neurological disability 2–3% per year.

Risk Factors for Haemorrhage

Size

Patients with small AVMs are more likely to present with haemorrhage than those with large AVMs. This is partly because small AVMs are less likely to cause seizures and progressive neurological deficit since a smaller cortical area is usually involved.

Graf et al. (1983) found that small size was an important risk factor for future haemorrhage of unruptured AVMs but only 12 of their patients had AVMs < 3 cm in diameter in their series. If the AVM had bled then the risk of rebleeding was not related to size (134 patients). Brown et al. (1988) did not find AVM size related to risk of bleeding for unruptured AVMs. The same findings were recently reported by Pollock et al. (1996). On the other hand, Spetzler et al. (1992) have measured the arterial pressure in feeding arteries to AVMs and found that the pressure in these arteries is higher in small AVMs and concluded that the risk of bleeding is higher. These findings were not confirmed by the work of Kader et al. (1994) who found only a weak correlation between nidal size and feed artery pressures Spetzler did find, however, that the size of haematoma resulting from haemorrhage of a small AVM was disproportionately large supporting his contention that small AVMs carry high risk of significant haemorrhage possibly due to greater arterial pressure.

Site

There is no consensus from the literature as to whether AVMs in any particular site have a higher risk from bleeding apart from those in the temporal lobe. Crawford et al. (1986) found that temporal lesions and to a lesser extent occipital lobe lesions were more likely to bleed than parietal lesions. Willinsky et al. (1988) also found that temporal lobe lesions were more likely to bleed. They found angiographic evidence of the draining veins being frequently obstructed by the free edge of the tentorium-cerebellum and the margin of the greater wing of sphenoid.

Lesions in the posterior fossa have a greater incidence of death from haemorrhage. Some authors believe that 50% of such haemorrhage are fatal, small volumes of blood capable causing brain stem compression.

Presentation

Haemorrhage

Are patients who harbour an AVM that has bled more likely to suffer further bleeds than those patients with other presentations? This is another controversial area. Whilst Samson and Barter (1991) in their review believe that there is little evidence that a history of previous haemorrhage is more likely to result in rebleed than patients without such a history, others disagree. Crawford calculated that 51% of her patients who presented with haemorrhage would have rebled at 20 years whereas for patients without a previous history of bleeding or epilepsy, the risk of rebleed was under 8%. More recently, Pollock et al. (1996) have reviewed, retrospectively, the histories of 315 patients specifically to look for risk factors that predict the bleeding risk of cerebral arteriovenous malformations. Using multivariate analysis they found a history of prior haemorrhage carried a relative risk of further haemorrhage of 9.0% with a 95% confidence interval 5.44–15.19.

These figures are convincing, despite the limitations of the study which was carried out on a highly selected group. On theoretical grounds if an AVM has become unstable and ruptured it is unlikely that the haematoma will alter the haemodynamic situation significantly except in the immediate situation and in the few cases where the nidus is partially obliterated by the bleed. Indeed, the bleed may result in a central false aneurysm, itself a risk factor. Further evidence that haemorrhage is indicative of haemodynamic instability comes from the greater risks of rehaemorrhage in the first year after initial bleed; six per cent of patients rebled in the first year in Graf's series and 18% in that of Fults'. Crawford also found that following a second haemorrhage from an AVM, the risk of further haemorrhage increased, adding weight to the theory that haemorrhage from an AVM is an indicator of haemodynamic instability. Recently Mast et al. (1997) has done a multivariate regression analysis on 281 AVMs followed up for 8.5 months. They found 17.8% annual risk of re-haemorrhage in the group that had presented with haemorrhage, whereas in the group that had presented without haemorrhage, it was only 2.2%. Interestingly, the rate of haemorrhage for men was three times that of women.

Haemorrhage in these studies has been defined as an event that is clinically symptomatic. MRI studies often show evidence of methaemaglobin and haemosiderin when no clinical event corresponding to a haemorrhage has been recorded. It is not known whether these patients who have not had symptoms of a haemorrhage have increased risk of rebleed or not. Unfortunately, spontaneous clotting and slow flow occurring in draining veins and in the nidus may also mimic the MR changes of a subclinical haemorrhage. Wilkins (1990) has given a clear definition of an presenting haemorrhage as one which is severe enough to lead to the diagnosis of an AVM in a patient who had previously not had such an episode. This remains the current definition.

Angioarchitecture

Arterial irregularity is common and may indicate abnormal structure but no clear-cut increased haemorrhagic risk has been shown for any of these arterial abnormalities apart from flow aneurysms (Willinsky et al., 1988; Crawford et al., 1986; Turjman et al., 1994).

Two *nidal* features increase the risk of haemorrhage of an AVM. A nidal aneurysm that is associated with a recent bleed, many of these aneurysms are false aneurysms with a wall of clot only (Turjman et al., 1994; Lasjaunian 1998). Secondly, the presence of fistulae increases the venous pressure and the risk of venous rupture. There is currently no consensus on the definition of a nidal fistula. Often, pragmatic definitions are used, e.g. the ability to pass a microcatheter into the venous side of the lesion. (Lundquist et al., 1996).

Miyasaka et al. (1992) analysed the *venous* system of AVMs and found three variable to correlate with increased risk of haemorrhage: a single draining vein, impaired venous drainage and deep venous drainage only. Venous stenosis and varices have been implicated as risk factors by Marks et al. (1990) and Willinsky et al. (1988).

Presenting Symptoms

Haemorrhage

Intracranial haemorrhage is the most devastating complications of an AVM. This may either result in a sudden neurological deficit or with the symptoms of subarachnoid haemorrhage. It is the initial presentation in at least 50% of cases. Children present in a similar way to adults but may also suffer cardiac failure if there is a high volume shunt and may rarely present with hydrocephalus. Recurrent haemorrhage is a strong indication for treatment as several authors have found that the chances of morbidity and death increases significantly with each recurrence.

Seizures

About a third of patients present with seizures. Lesions close to the Rolandic fissure are particularly likely to present with seizures. Several authors have noted an increased risk of haemorrhage after seizure (Graf et al., 1983; Crawford et al., 1986). Others have found that the mode of presentation did not affect outcome (Brown et al., 1988; Ondra et al., 1990).

Neurological Deficit

About 10% of patients present with neurological deficit. This typically presents with cognitive deficit and particularly with memory problems. However, some patients develop gradual weakness or visual loss.

Treatment of AVMs

Surgery

The Risks and Benefits of Surgery

Recently, several authors have stated that the results of surgery for small AVMs or AVMs in the Spetzler–Martin grade 1–2 are so good that other treatment is not indicated (Spetzler, 1997) and indeed it may be unethical (Heros, 1997). It is, therefore, important to analyse these published surgical results so that fair comparison with other treatment modalities and with the natural history can be made.

For small AVMs the recent results obtained by microsurgery are indeed impressive. Sundt et al. presented a series of 242 patients treated by microsurgery. The mortality rate was 0%, permanent neurological deficit was 4.4% (Sundt et al., 1991). Similar results were obtained by Sisti et al. (1993) of his 67 patients only one suffered permanent neurological deficit. Yasargil's series (1987b) is the largest published; for the 414 patients the mortality was 0.8% with a permanent disability of 5.1%. For a subgroup of smaller AVMs less than 4 cm in size in his series the mortality was 0.8%. Most recently Schuller and Schramn (1997) have produced similar figures with a 4.8% permanent disability, of which only 3.2% were considered significant. The disinterested clinician, however, needs to look very closely at these results. The authors exclude any deficits that could be expected from surgery, e.g. visual field deficits from occipital AVMs. There was considerable non-neurological surgical morbidity (9.7%) and the average hospital stay was 24 days. Only 70% of patients achieved independence and 10% remained severely disabled. This considerable non-surgical morbidity that occurs in treating the most surgically accessible and smallest AVMs is likely to be greater in the larger AVMs and is not seen with the other modalities of treatment.

The morbidity of surgery increases with Spetzler–Martin grade. Spetzler and Martin's (1986) group encountered major morbidity in 4% of grade 3 patients, 7% of grade 4 and 12% of grade 5. Heros (1990) likewise achieved only a 63% good outcome (or better in grade 5 patients.

The published surgical results are those from enthusiastic centres. Such is the nature of surgical research it has recently prompted an eminent British neurosurgeon to compare the ever improving results to the world 100 metres spring record; this is always being broken, but the rest of us are not running any faster.

A more dispassionate look at the results of surgery has been undertaken by Chadwick and Crawford (1990). They cite the American Co-operative Study (Perret 1966) as being more representative of the complication rate of the average centre (Foster, 1997). The immediate mortality was 10%. The morbidity for their own patients (Crawford et al., 1986) was a 65% risk of neurological deficit over 20 years follow up for ruptured AVMs excised compared to a 42% risk of deficit if conservatively managed. Likewise, 20% of surgical patients lost their independence by the time of discharge compared with 5% amongst those conservatively managed. It could be argued that modern techniques are likely to have changed these figures but interestingly that was not the experience of Crawford. The passage of time, 1970-1986, had no effect on either the morbidity or the mortality of surgery for patients presenting with haemorrhage. Van Gynn (1996) has recently reviewed the surgical data and concluded that even in carefully selected patients the serious permanent morbidity is in the order of 8%.

In summary, there are few areas of medicine which are in greater need for a prospective trial with randomization of patients.

Radiosurgery

Initial results with non-fractionated whole brain radiation were poor (Laing et al., 1992). But two methods have since evolved for delivering a more focused dose of radiotherapy. The "gamma knife", which utilizes multiple cobalt sources that are placed into a helmet around the head and the "linnac", which uses a neutron beam produced by a linear accelerator. This beam is concentrated on the AVM typically using a polycycloidal motion this ensures that the dose to the surrounding brain is kept to a minimum.

Both methods require the head to be firmly fixed. This is either achieved by pins screwed into the skull vault or by using a mouth plate individually modelled to the patient's upper palate. Neither method is pleasant for the patient, and frequently we administer morphine (10 mg) to patients who are undergoing angiography in the stereotactic frame.

The Results of Radiosurgery

The early results for stereotactic radiosurgery were encouraging. Lunsford et al. (1991) obliterated 83% of AVMs with a diameter of 2.5 cm or less in 67 patients with a low morbidity of 2-3%. There is a long time of 1-2 years before obliteration is complete and risks of bleeding during this period range from 0 to 16% with an average of 7%. Schaller and Schramm (1997) have published an overview of the radiosurgical series. Those authors using the Linnac or the gamma knife technology achieved a 71-84% obliteration rate for small AVMs when assessed by DSA with a morbidity of 0-13% from radionecrosis, with most series reporting 3-5% morbidity. Local cerebral oedema is quite a frequent complication, occurring in up to 23% in Lunford's series (Lunsford et al., 1991) but typically it responds to steroids. When the AVM was greater than 2.5 cm in diameter the obliteration rate was markedly less – in the region of 58-46%. Likewise, the incidence of neurological deficits following radiosurgery also increases with size of the AVM being irradiated.

Interventional Radiology

Embolisation of AVMs was first attempted in the 1980s and evolved with the development of microcatheters (Luessenhap & Rosa, 1984). Originally, particles of gelfoam or fragments impregnated with isopropyl alcohol were flushed through the catheter. Although these agents were useful, particularly prior to surgery, they have been replaced with agents that lead to permanent occlusion of vessels and which can also form a cast of the AVM. The most popular of these are forms of cyanoacrylate, a rapidly polymerising liquid glue.

The field is rapidly evolving, with new catheter systems that regularly enter the nidus and new embolisation agents which allow for more control during injection.

Practical Considerations of Embolisation

Anaesthesia
This will depend on the angioarchitecture and the patient. If the nidus can be easily reached with the microcatheter then the chances of embolisation, with reflux back into normal vessels, is very small and the procedure is then more easily performed under general anaesthesia (GA). This is particularly true for young patients (under 12 years) and old patients who may find procedural times of several hours most uncomfortable. Typically, the radiologist is uncertain prior to intervention that the nidus will be reached and that all the vessels requiring to be embolised do not also supply normal brain, as these branches sometimes only become apparent when several of the main feeders have been obliterated. Some information can be obtained from the MRI particularly if the AVM can be seen to lie in a sulcus; these sulcal AVM's can usually be embolised safely under GA. Some patients will already have had an exploratory selective angiogram to establish whether a safe catheter position can be achieved. Again these patients may have a GA but for the majority of patients neuroleptic anaesthesia is used. In our department either propofol or madazolam are administered by an anesthetist. Both drugs provide anaesthesia that is rapidly reversible and allow sodium amytal testing (see below). These drugs potentially depress respiration and may induce a breathing pattern that leads to considerable head movement making subtraction angiography problematical. The PO_2 should be monitored to prevent hypoxia occurring; CO_2 retention is not usually a problem unless airway obstruction occurs.

The Coaxial System
Guide Catheter A typical coaxial system consists of a wide bore 6F guide catheter through which passes a microcatheter. The most useful guides have a soft tip, which has a small hockey-stick curve. This assists selection of the internal carotid artery and then advancement to the petrous segment of the internal carotid artery without intimal damage. Such distal placement results in a firm platform for microcatheters which otherwise can push the guide catheter back into the aorta when they encounter tortuous distal vessels. In elderly patients or those with tortuous carotid arteries, the carotid is selected using a catheter specifically shaped for the anatomy e.g. Simmons type III catheter and then the guide is exchanged over a long exchange guide wire. The techniques for using these catheters have recently been detailed by Morris (1997), whose book is an excellent practical guide.

Haemostatic Valve and Flush These valves are extremely simple but highly effective pieces of equipment. A rubber "doughnut" is inserted within a perspex sleeve. As the distal end is screwed on the rubber is compressed with its central hole reducing in diameter. This allows for a variety of microcatheters to be introduced and manipulated whilst maintaining a water-tight seal. Recently, Nycomed have introduced new haemostatic valves that do not require unscrewing to enable penetration.

There is typically a side arm connected to the perspex sleeve of a haemostatic valve, this allows heparinised flush to pass between the microcatheter and the guide, reducing friction and preventing the catheter from clotting. A three-way valve introduced into the flush tubing permits contrast injections to be performed as necessary. It is extremely important to check that the tubing, the taps and the valves are free of air. Air embolus may result in stroke. Occasionally, valve systems are partially airtight and prior to any injection through the system we habitually check that no air has entered by very gently withdrawing into the syringe; this will usually detects any leaks.

Microcatheters The technology of microcatheters is rapidly evolving and is the main reason why recent endovascular series of document such improvement in terms of success of AVM obliteration and reduced morbidity. The two basic types of microcatheter are those that are wire directed and those that are flow directed. This distinction, however, is becoming blurred as wires are now small enough to be used with flow directed catheters giving them some steerability. Flow-directed catheters can be manipulated by flushing with small volumes of saline (Turjman et al., 1994). Both types of catheter will frequently travel around bends more easily if the tip have been previously steamed into a curve. We use wire-directed catheters when the main flow from the distal internal carotid is not to the AVM, taking a flow-directed catheter away from the AVM. This is often the case when the AVM is fed by perforators, or is small. Many makes are currently now available including the Tracker catheter (Boston Scientific) and Prowler catheter (Cordis). Each catheter has slightly different properties and often in difficult cases a variety will usually be tried. It is recommend that the operator becomes familiar with one system and then tries other types in difficult circumstances – there is little consensus as to which system is superior. Several manufacturers have now introduced braided catheters. This increases stiffness and the catheter can be forced more distally, but care not to perforate fragile vessels must be taken.

The "magic" catheter designed by Moret and Balt has long been the standard flow-directed catheter. The distal segment of up to 30 cm is made of pursil, a very floppy plastic that allows the catheter to be carried by arterial blood flow towards and into the nidus. We have found the thinner 1.5F diameter catheters can be too closely wrapped to the arterial wall and be difficult to retrieve and occasionally fracture. Although this has not resulted in complications we prefer the 1.8F system. Recently Target, Cordis and MIS have produced flow-directed catheters and we are currently doing comparative testing of this new generation of catheters.

Indications for Embolisation

Preoperative Embolisation

Embolisation is frequently used as an adjunct to surgery for AVMs. The risks of surgery appear to be directly related to size (Spetzler & Martin, 1986) and although complete obliteration of an AVM may not be possible by embolisation, surgery can be made technically far easier following partial obliteration. Not only is the flow is reduced and blood loss minimised but the dangers of perfusion breakthrough are also decreased. This phenomenon occurs in a small group of patients (Vinuela, 1992) when the blood flow to the AVM is redirected by surgery to normal tissues unused to high blood flow and pressure. Severe oedema and haemorrhage can result.

Technique

Although reduction in size of the nidus is important, it is obliteration of the deep arterial feeders that is often of most value to the surgeon. The deep perforating arteries and the occipital arteries are usually the most difficult to control surgically, but consultation with the surgeon concerned is essential prior to the procedure. The gluing technique, likewise, may be altered for presurgical embolisation so that a short arterial cast is formed rather than gluing the venous outflow with its dangers. Surgery is performed at 10-14 days, after which time thrombosis is complete. After 2 weeks a florid neovascularity can surround the AVM formed by leptomeningeal collaterals that make surgery difficult. Surprisingly, vessels that are occluded with glue are soft and can easily cut (Vinuela, 1992a).

One situation that can lead to bleeding is the obstruction of a single venous outflow tract without obliteration of one of the arterial feeders. Sluggish venous flow and evidence of stasis is an indication for considering immediate surgery (Figure 5.5).

Results of Embolisation Prior to Surgery

The results of embolisation prior to surgery have been mixed. Jaffar et al. (1993) have compared two groups, one of which went for surgery following embolisation, the other without prior embolisation. The 20 patients who were embolised had a 15% incidence of haemorrhage and a 5% incidence of transient ischaemia resulting from the embolisation. The operative and postoperative complications were not statistically different in both groups and neither was the long-term outcome. Since the group was small (only 13 patients in the non-embolised group) inferences from this study must be guarded but the authors did conclude that since the AVMs that were embolized were larger (3.9 cm mean diameter compared with 2.3 cm of those not embolised) embolisation was of value. The results of Deruty et al. (1993) of a larger group of patients treated with a multidisciplinary approach were less encouraging. Of their 67 patients, 28% deteriorated as a result of embolisation treatment. All the complications following surgery or radiotherapy remained minor but of those cases that were embolised this caused deterioration in 25%. Although the deficit was minor in 13%, death occurred in 8% and a neurological deficit in 5%. Clearly, preoperative embolisation has significant risks and should not be undertaken without clear cut goals.

Embolisation Prior to Radiosurgery

Many studies have shown that the efficacy of radiosurgery is markedly reduced for AVMs with a nidal diameter of greater than 3 cm (Schaller & Schramm, 1997). Other angiographic features that indicate poor outcome from radiotherapy have recently been identified (Meder et al.). The presence of high flow shunts in the nidus reduces the chances of obliteration with radiosurgery. Embolisation can occlude the fistulae and reduce the size of AVMs improving the chances of obliteration of the AVM by radiosurgery. In addition, if there are high risk clinical or angiographic features present, such as nidal (false) aneurysms then embolisation may be indicated to stabilise a situation since radiotherapy frequently takes up two years to obliterate an AVM.

Embolisation technique is similar to that employed prior to surgery except that the aim is usually to penetrate and obliterate the nidus, whereas the surgeon may be more interested in purely the obliteration of surgically inaccessible arterial feeders. It is important to try and assess, prior to setting out on the path of embolisation, whether it is possible to reduce the size of the AVM. Frequently, embolisation succeeds in simply "splattering" the AVM, taking out small central areas of the nidus without reducing the total volume that requires irradiation. Such a result simply exposes the patient to the increased risk of embolisation without reducing the risks of radiosurgery. It is difficult to predict the results of embolisation but the presence of multiple feeders and small feeders supplying a large AVM which is multi-compartmental and deep, are all features that make embolisation in this context unlikely to be successful.

The Results of Embolisation Combined with Radiosurgery

There are no good figures to show that partial embolisation reduces the risk of bleeding before stereotactic radiation has eliminated the AVM, apart from the data from the Karolinska Hospital (Lundquist et al., 1990). Lundquist found that for large AVMs, partial embolisation increased the risk over the natural history. Both Lasjaunias and Picard (personal communication) believe that partial embolisation does reduce the risk of bleeding when comparing their embolised patients with their own controls, i.e. patients not suitable for surgery and carrying perhaps a higher risk of bleeding than is normally quoted. In summary, although the jury is still out over whether partial embolisation reduces the risk of haemorrhage, what is certain is that embolisation can reduce the volume and diameter of an AVM, making it suitable for surgery or radiotherapy.

Endovascular Obliteration of AVMs

Indications

Small AVMs (less than 4 cm) with less than three feeders and with few compartments and draining veins are those most likely to be obliterated (Figure 5.2). Sulcal AVMs fed by end arteries are more easily treated than deep or gyral AVMs which often have transit arteries.

Technique

The first state of embolisation is frequently an *endovascular arterial exploration*. The aim of this is to establish the following:

1. Is this *AVM likely to be obliterated by embolisation* and is access to the nidus possible with microcatheters? Is the AVM sulcal or gyral (Figure 5.3).
2. What is the *angioarchitecture*?

To assess risk factors including the presence of fistulae and false aneurysms that should be treated first and to assess the venous outflow – if there is a single venous outflow this should be blocked with the last glue injection to prevent rupture (Fig. 5.2b).

A coaxial system is used with a guide catheter positioned in the internal carotid. Flow-directed or wire-directed catheters may be used to select feeders. Small feeders that have lesser flow will often require a catheter directed by a wire. Patience is a virtue in negotiating tortuous vessels, but with modern catheters most nidal areas can eventually be reached.

Sodium Amytal

If the nidus is not reached then we routinely use sodium amytal (30–50 mg) before embolising a feeder. The amytal is given in conjunction with testing to appropriate

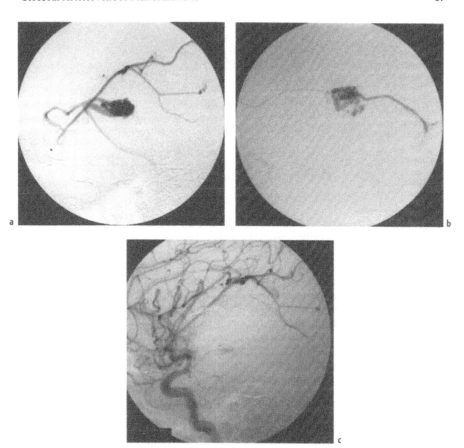

Fig. 5.2. Left temporal AVM. **a** Selective DSA reveals a small AVM with one main feeder and no transit arteries. **b** Catheterization of the nidus with a wire directed catheter required since main flow was to the posterior paretal artery. **c** Check angiography reveals complete obliteration of AVM.

neurology for the area of brain involved. It is important that prior to testing that the neuroleptic anaesthesia (propofol) is sufficiently reversed to have a co-operative patient. More subtle brain ischaemia may be picked up by performing the amytal test in conjunction with EEG recording (Ranch et al., 1992). If a feeding artery to normal brain is identified many are reluctant to embolise despite negative amytal test as these "silent" areas of the brain may later result in changes in personality (Van Gynn, 1996).

Glue Technique

Gluing techniques of AVMs differ around the world. Two main techniques are uses, one that advocates using high concentrations of glue mixed with lipoidal, e.g. 1:1/2, the other that uses much more diluted glue 1:3 or 1:4 to lipoidal. The second type of injection achieves further penetration of the nidus but typically involves a longer injection time and higher risks of venous embolisation and catheter tip sticking to the vessels. If using very dilute glue a useful technique is to start by extruding a very

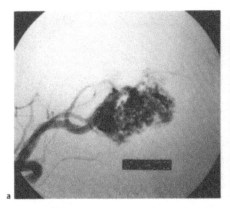
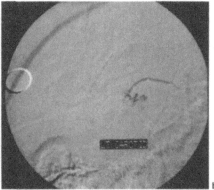

Fig. 5.3. A large left temporal AVM. **a** Non-selective DSA injection. **b** Selective DSA shows the AVM supplied by a transit artery that also supplies normal cortex. This is typical of a gyral type of AVM. The chances of successful obliteration by interventional radiology are small.

small bubble of glue; this is allowed to set for a few seconds then is slowly pushed through the nidus. Compartments may open during such a slow push. The injection is stopped when venous penetration is achieved or if significant reflux occurs.

The microcatheters occasionally become fixed in the glue. Typically attempts at withdrawal lead to a distal fracturing of the catheter. This is sometimes associated with local haemorrhage. Surprisingly, the incidence of subsequent death or major disability is low (Van Halbach et al., 1991). Modern catheters (e.g. Spinnaker) are coated so as to resist being glued into vessels and much longer injection times (up to 2 minutes) are becoming more popular. The presence of rapid shunts within a nidus may prompt the use of combination techniques including coils, balloons or nearly neat glue (Figures 5.4 and 5.5) as well as using more dilute glue for slower flow areas.

Other Embolic Agent

There has been a great deal of experience with histoacryl but its very rapid setting times (sometimes 0.2 seconds from injection) can lead to problems with rapid reflux in normal vessels. Hence there has been a search for materials that have better control. Ethibloc has achieved considerable acceptance in Germany. It can be squeezed into the AVM like a toothpaste, although it is awkward to prepare. Others have used alcohol or particles. Particles are generally safer than glue as they do not penetrate small unseen anastamoses but typically lead to only a temporary occlusion of an AVM feeder. Hence, they are more commonly used as an adjunct to surgery. More recently a copolymer Embolyx has been used to occlude AVMs. This is dissolved in DMSO which itself is toxic if injected fast and dissolves intradural catheter plastics. It does however allow long (up to 5 minutes) injections without risk of catheter fracture.

Complications from Embolisation of AVMs

The complication rate is exceptionally difficult to assess, with results ranging from a complication rate of 0.5% mortality and 1.5% severe morbidity for 188 patients in the New York University series of patients. At the other end of the spectrum is a series of 53 consecutive patients in whom 5 died and 17 had permanent deficit (Van Gynn,

Cerebral Arteriovenous Malformations

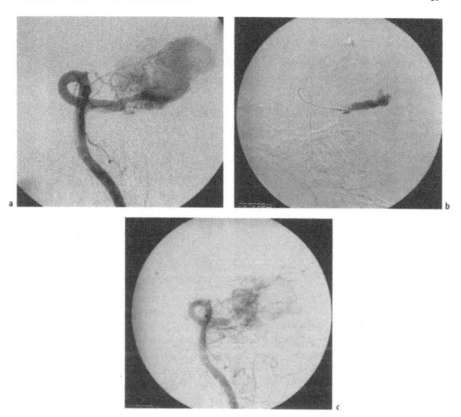

Fig. 5.4. a Posterior cerebral artery fistula revealed by DSA. b Caliberated balloon used with high concentration glue mixture. c Post-embolization with a glue cast of the feeding vessel.

1996). Frizzell, reviewing the world literature of over 1200 patients, found an 8% complication rate from AVM embolisation. This figure almost certainly suffers from publication bias and few small centres or centres with poor figures are unlikely to publish their results. These figures do, however, concur with those of one of the most respected figures in endovascular treatment, Vinuela, whose 283 patients had a 28% immediate complication rate with a 13% long-term neurological deficit and 2.5% death rate (Vinuela, 1992b). However, most of his deaths occurred when using calibrated leak balloon technique and were due to haemorrhage following over-inflation of the balloon. More recently, the Gotenborg group from Sweden have shown that with improving techniques the morbidity and mortality figures could be substantially improved. Of a group of 150 patients treated from 1987–1993 the overall complication rate was high (40%) of which 6.7% were severe, but in the last year (Masko et al., 1990) none had severe complications or died. The ability to penetrate the nidus with microcatheters certainly reduced the complication rate and the chances of obliteration. It is a very difficult to compare these complication rates with an equivalent surgical series over 85% of the Gotenborg patients were Spetzler grade 3 or worse. When suitable AVMs are selected for embolisation, a 65% obliteration rate can be achieved (Muller Farrel & Valvarius, 1995; Valvaris, 1998) with very low mortality (1.3%) and low

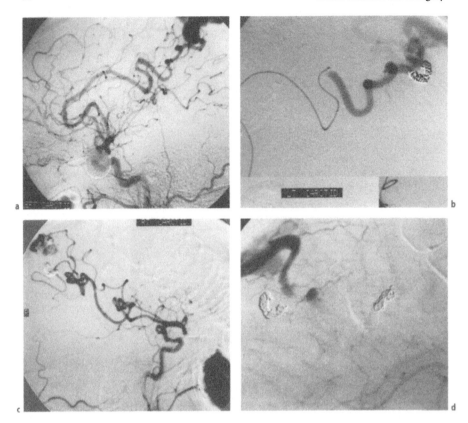

Fig. 5.5. **a** Left carotid angiogram demonstrating a peripheral parietal AVM with a large fistulous component. **b** Fistula partly occluded by coil embolization. **c** Right carotid angiogram demonstrating nidal filling possible due to angiogenesis. **d** Late venous phase reveals early clot formation in the draining vein. Venous obstructed led to a small cortical haemorrhage with transient symptoms.

morbidity: 1.3% severe, 1.5% moderate, 2.3% mild residual deficit. Our own complications have come from two situations reflux of glue into transit arteries (Figure 5.3) or from venous thrombosis/occlusion to the outflow of an AVM when the feed arteries of that compartment have not been completely obliterated (Figure 5.5)

Treatment of AVMs in Special Situations

Early Treatment of AVMs Following Haemorrhage

Early surgical management of AVMs is restricted to those cases in which the mass effect of the haemotoma is life threatening. Operating on a swollen brain is not technically easy.

We have recently treated a series of 10 patients with endovascular intervention in the acute phase (day 2–7) following haemorrhage. Seven of these patients had complete obliteration at 6 months follow up. One patient suffered temporary deterioration. Rodesh et al. (1992) has also reported three cases successfully treated acutely. Patients particularly at risk from early rebleeding, such as those with false aneurysms, are suitable for early treatment. It is also worth considering for patients who are severely immobilized by the haemorrhage and deep venous thrombosis can be anticipated. There is a risk of early rebleeding; 6% of Graf's patients rebled in the first year (Graf et al., 1983). Early embolisation also redistributes the blood flow and may reduce the ischaemia surrounding the haematoma by reducing venous hypertension and increasing local perfusion. Finally, compression of the nidus may have contributed to our high success rate of complete obliteration.

Treatment for AVMs Presenting with Seizures

It has frequently been argues that treatment of AVMs presenting with seizures should be more conservative. There is little, however, in the literature to support this view. Ondra et al. (1990) found in his prospective review of AVM patients that the yearly mortality of 1% was not affected by mode of presentation. In Crawford's series the incidence of bleeding in a patient presenting with seizures was less than that of patients who presented with haemorrhage; but over a 10-year period it was only 26% when compared with 42%, but the problems with this paper have already been documented (Crawford et al., 1986).

Reduction of Seizures by Embolisation and by Other Modalities

Several authors have shown good results for surgical excision in curing and reducing seizures. Piepgras reported on 270 AVM patients operated on who also had seizures. 89% of these were seizure free at 2 years (Piepgras et al., 1993). Yeh obtained similar results with only one out of 54 patients operated on left with seizures that were not cured (Yeh et al., 1993). A cautionary note was struck by Crawford who found that in her last series the chances of developing epilepsy were substantially increased by surgery. (Crawford et al., 1986). The results of embolisation for epilepsy have been less impressive. Lundquist found that the epilepsy of only 35% of his patients was improved despite many of these patients having supplementary surgery. Lasjaunias and Berenstein (1987) found that 91 of 134 patients with seizures were free of seizures after embolisation but noted that many of these patients may have been improved by proper medication in a controlled hospital environment. Neither radiosurgery nor embolisation removes gliotic tissue surrounding the AVM; indeed radiosurgery, and to a lesser extent embolisation, may induce gliosis. Forster (1997) presented a series of 149 patients who had had at least one seizure in the year prior to radiosurgery. 54% had no seizures up to 4 years after radiosurgery (averages 2-year follow-up).

Decision Making in the Management of AVMs

As will have become clear, it is often not the actual treatment that requires the most skill in managing AVMs but deciding whether to treat it at all. Often the evidence from the literature is conflicting. Which method of treatment to recommend can be an even more difficult decision in the absence of any controlled data.

This section is a synopsis of what we tell our patients and why. It is one of the mysteries of medicine that after long discussions with two patients about how to treat two apparently similar vascular lesions, one can end up with two very different conclusions about best management. The patient's response to the information given is a crucial factor in the final decisions.

Risks of Doing Nothing

We tell patients that the risk of haemorrhage from their AVM is 4% per year and that the risk of this resulting in a neurological deficit is 2.7% per year with a risk of death of 1% per year (Ondra et al., 1990). These figures are similar to those of the study by Ondra but are slightly higher than those of Brown (Brown et al., 1988) and Crawford et al. (1986). We explain that it is a cumulative risk and show those who have a better understanding of mathematics the calculations done by Kondiziolka et al. (1995) (Table 5.2).

Table 5.2. Risk of haemorrhage from an AVM

Age at presentation	Years to live	Risk of haemorrhage at 2%/yr (%)	Risk of haemorrhage at 4%/yr (%)
0	76	79	96
15	62	71	92
25	52	65	88
35	43	58	83
45	34	50	75
55	25	40	64
65	18	31	52
75	11	20	36
85	6	11	22

From Kondiziolka et al., 1995.

Presentation

We are not yet convinced that mode of presentation makes a significant difference to the long term outlook for patients with AVMs. Both in the study by Ondra et al. (1990) and that of Brown et al. (1988), the long-term follow-up of patients with other presentations other than that of haemorrhage, indicated that the morbidity and mortality of patients was not significantly affected by presentation. It does however seem likely that an initial presentation with haemorrage paradoxically predicts a higher chance of further bleeds (are these bleeds confined by gliosis?).

It is however logical to think of a new haemorrhage as an indicator that the AVM has become unstable. Graf found that AVMs had a 6% rebleed (Graf et al., 1983) rate in the first year and Mast et al. (1997) recently found that 17% of patients who presented with haemorrhage rebled within a year. We suggest early treatment for patients who have clinical evidence of having recently bled particularly when careful angiography reveals a nidal aneurysm. There are some advantages of both operating and embolising the AVM in the subacute phase of the illness (2-7 days). This is particularly true if the patient is immobilised by the ictus and at risk from thromboembolism. If evidence for haemorrhage is confined to the MRI changes only, it is ignored, as it is felt that methaemoglobin and haemosiderin could result from spontaneous thrombosis of parts of the nidus and venous drainage.

Treatment Strategy

No Treatment

If the patient is old and not developing a progressive neurological deficit, we will not recommend any treatment other than symptomatic management. AVMs that are larger than 6 cm with multiple feeders as well as those deeply situated can seldom be cured and all modalities of treatment will also carry an unjustifiably high morbidity.

Active Treatment

Stage 1
For all AVMs in our unit, the first stage of treatment is to have a microangiographic endovascular exploration. This details the angioarchitecture and helps to quantify the risks of each of the possible treatments.

If clear treatment aims can be established then embolisation is frequently carried out as well at this stage with modern catheters and techniques it is often possible to achieve quickly a safe intranidal position.

Stage 2
It is usually possible after the first embolisation to have a very good idea as to whether the lesion is likely to be obliterated endovascularly. This is the first option, as it is now considered the least invasive method of treatment. If the architecture mitigates against embolisation, further consultation is undertaken and further embolisation is only undertaken if it is thought that the lesion could be made suitable for surgery or stereotactic radiosurgery. The radiologist should be aware of precisely which vessels the surgeon is likely to have difficulty clipping and what is required to make the lesion suitable for radiosurgery. Small lesions will often not require further embolisation.

Stage 3: Surgery or Radiosurgery
Surgery has the advantage of being potentially able to achieve an immediate "cure" of the AVM. This is attractive for small superficial lesions in non-eloquent areas. The risks of surgery are assessed by using the Spetzler–Martin scale but each AVM needs to be individually assessed by the neurosurgeon.

Radiosurgery To the morbidity of radiosurgery (5%) must be added the 3–5% morbidity related to haemorrhage from the AVM during the 2 years that radiosurgery typically takes to complete by obliterating the lesion. In our institution, radiosurgery is used if the lesion does not fit into the above categories. Although deep lesions also respond poorly to radiosurgery, we have found it a very successful method of treating AVMs that have been reduced to under 3 cm in size.

Over the past 2 years, 30% of patients have been treated by embolisation alone, 10% by surgery alone, 20% by radiosurgery alone. 10% by embolisation and surgery and 40% by embolisation and radiosurgery.

Treatment Costs and Patient Preference

The treatment costs of a ruptured AVM depend largely on the rate and severity of the bleed. Our centre offers all three modalities of treatment at the costs shown in Table 5.3 for unruptured AVMs.

Table 5.3. Costs of different treatment modalities

Modality	Cost (£)
Radiotherapy (linnac)	3000
Surgery	3500
Endovascular embolisation	1500 (per session)

Patient preference has been for the endovascular method of treatment. Some patients find the oral plate and stereotactic frame very uncomfortable. Those having gamma knife treatment require the frame to be fixed to the skull with screws. Surgery is the least preferred option by most patients.

References

Anderson IB, Peterson J, Mortensen EL et al. (1988) Conservatively treated patients with cerebral arteriovenous malformation; mental and physical outcome. 51: 1208-1212

Brown RD, Weibers DO, Forbes G et al. (1988) The natural history of unruptured intracranial arteriovenous malformations. J Neurosurgery 68: 352-357

Crawford PM, West CR, Chadwick DW (1986) Arteriovenous malformations of the brain, natural history in unoperated patients. JNNP 49: 1-10

Deruty R, Pelissou-Guyotat I, Mottolese C, Bascoulergue Y, Amat D (1993) The combined management of cerebral arteriovenous malformations. Experience with 100 cases and review of the literature. Acta Neurochir 123 (3-4): 101-112

Forster D (1997) Results of radiosurgery for brain arteriovenous malformations. Presented at the Brain Interface Meeting, Birmingham, UK, 1997

Frizzel RT, Fisher WS (1995) Cure, morbidity, and mortality associated with embolization of brain arteriovenous malformations: a review of 1246 patients. J Neurosurg 37(b): 1031-9

Fults P, Kelly DC (1984) Natural history of arteriovenous malformations of the brain – a clinical study. Neurosurgery 15: 658-662

Graf CT, Peret GE, Torner JC (1983) Bleeding from cerebral arteriovenous malformations as part of their natural history. J Neurosurgery 58: 331-337

Heros RC (1997) Comment on microsurgical AVM therapy. Neurosurgery 40: 672-673

Houdart E, Gobin YP, Cassaco A et al. (1993) A proposed angiographic classification of intra cranial arteriovenous fistulae malformations Neuroradiology 35: 381-385

Jafar JJ, Davis AJ, Berenstein A, Choi IS, Kupersmith MJ (1993) The effect of embolization with N-butyl cyanoacrylate prior to surgical resection of cerebral arteriovenous malformations. J Neurosurgery 78(1): 60-69

Jellinger K (1986) Vascular malformations of the ventral nervous system: a morphological overview. Neurosurg Rev 9: 177-216

Kader A, Young WC, Pice-Speckman J et al. (1994) The influence of haemodynamic and anatomic factors on haemorrhage from cerebral arteriovenous malformations. Neurosurgery 34: 801-808

Kondziolka D, McLaughlin MR, Kestle JRW (1995) Simple risk predictions for arteriovenous malformation haemorrhage. Neurosurgery 37: 851-855

Laing RW, Childs J, Brada M (1992) Failure of conventionally fractioned radiotherapy to decrease the risk of haemorrhage in unoperated arteriovenous malformations. Neurosurgery 30: 872-878

Lasjaunias P (1998) Angioarchitecture of 500 arteriovenous malformations. Presented at the Interventional Workshop Val D'Isere, 1998

Lasjaunias B, Berenstein A (1987) Surgical neuro angiography, Vol 2. Springer Verlag, New York, p 131

Luessenthopp AJ, Rosa C (1984) Cerebral arteriovenous malformations; indications for and results of surgery and the role of intra-vascular techniques. J Neurosurgery 60: 14-22

Lundquist C, Wikholm G, Svendsen P (1996) Embolization of cerebral arteriovenous malformations Part II – aspects of complications and late outcome. Neurosurgery 39: 460-467

Lunsford CD, Kondziolka D, Flickinger JC et al. (1991) Stereotactic radiosurgery for arteriovenous malformations of the brain. J Neurosurg 75: 512-524

Marks MP, Lane B, Steinburg GK et al. (1990) Haemorrhage in intracerebral arteriovenous malformations: angiographic determinants. Radiology 176: 807-813

Mast H, Young WC, Keonnecke HC et al. (1997) Risk of spontaneous haemorrahage after diagnosis of cerebral arteriovenous malformation. Lancet 350: 1065-1068

McCormick WF (1962) The pathology of vascular arteriovenous malformations. J Neurosurg 24 (7): 807-816

Meder JF, Openheim C, Blustajn J. Cerebral arteriovenous malformations: the value of radiologic parameters in predicting response to radiosurgery. AJNR 18: 1473-1483

Miyasaka Y, Yada K, Ohwada T et al. (1992) The analysis of venous drainage as a factor in haemorrhage from arteriovenous malformations. J Neurosurgery 16: 239-243

Morris P (1997) Practical neuroangiography. Williams & Wilkins, Baltimore

Muller Forrel W, Valavanis A (1995) How angioarchitecture of cerebral arteriovenous malformations should influence therapeutic considerations. Min Inv Neurosurg 38: 32-40

Ondra SC, Troupp H, George ED et al. (1990) The natural history of symptomatic arteriovenous malformations of the brain: a 24 year follow up assessment. J Neurosurgery 73: 387-391

Petereit D, Metha M, Turski P et al. (1993) Treatment of arteriovenous malformations with stereotactic radiosurgery employing both magnetic resonance angiography and standard angiography as a data base. Int J Radiat Oncol Biol Phys 25: 309-313

Piepgras DG, Dundt TM Jnr, Kagoorwanski AT, Stevens AL (1993) Seizure outcome in patients with surgically treated cerebral arteriovenous malformations. J Neurosurgery 78(1): 5-11

Pollock BE, Flickinger JC, Lunsford CD et al. (1996) Factors that predict bleeding risk of cerebral arteriovenous malformations. Stroke 1: 1-6

Rauch RA, Vinuela F, Duckwiler G (1992) Pre-embolization functional evaluation in brain arteriovenous malformations: the ability of superselective amytal test to predict neurologist dysfunction before embolization. AJNR 13(1): 309-314

Rodesch G, Parker F, Garcia M (1992) The role of embolization in the emergency treatment of ruptured cerebral arteriovenous malformations. Neurochirgie 38(s): 282-290

Samson D, Batjer HH (1991) Pre-operative evaluation of the risk/benefit ratio for artervenous malformations of the brain. In: Wilkins RH, Rengachary SS (eds) Neurosurgery update II. McGraw-Hill, New York, NY pp 129-133

Schaller C, Schramm J (1997) Micro-surgical results for small arteriovenous malformations accessible for radiosurgical or embolization. Neurosurgery 40(4): 664-672

Sisti MB, Kader A, Stein BM (1993) Microsurgery for 67 intracranial arteriovenous malformations less than 3 cm in diameter. J Neurosurgery 79: 653-660

Spetzler R (1997) Arteriovenous malformations. Presented at the 3rd International Congress of Minimally Invasive Neurosurgery, Paris 1997.

Spetzler RF, Martin NA (1986) A proposed grading system for grading intra-cranial arteriovenous malformations. J Neurosurgery 65: 476-483

Spetzler RF, Hargraves RW, McCormick PW, et al. (1992) Relationship of perfusion pressure and size to risk of haemorrhage from AVMs. J Neurosurgery 76: 918-923

Sundt TM, Peipgras DG, Stevens CN (1991) Surgery for supratentorial arteriovenous malformations in clinical neurosurgery. Proceedings of the Congress of Neurological Surgeons 1989. Williams & Williams, Baltimore, pp 46-115

Theron J, Newton TH, Hoyt WF (1974) Unilateral retinocephalic vascular malformations. Neuroradiology 7: 185-196

Turjman FT, Massoud TF, Vinuela F et al. (1994) Aneurysms related to cerebal artriovenous malformations: superselective angioraphic assessment in 58 patients. AJNR 15: 1601-1605

Valavanis A (1998) The James Bull Lecture. British Society of Neuroradiology, Cork, 1998

Van Gynn J (1996) In Warlow CP (ed) Stroke, Blackwell, Oxford, pp 469-476

Van Halbach V, Higashida RT, Dowd CF et al. (1991) Management of vascular perforations that occur during neuro-interventional procedures. AJNR 12: 319-327

Vinuela F (1992a) Interventional neuroradiology. Raven Press, New York, pp 77-87

Vinuela F (1992b) Functional evaluation and embolization of intracranial arteriovenous malformations in interventional neuroradiology. In: Vinuela F, Halbach V U, Dion J E (Eds) Raven Press, New York pp 77-87

Wilkins RH (1990) Natural history of brain AVMs in intracranial vascular malformations. American Association of Neurological Surgeons, Illinois pp 31-34

Willinsky R, Lasjaunias P, Terbrugge K, Pruvost P (1988) Brain arteriovenous malformations: analysis of the angioarchitecture in relationship to haemorrhage. J Neuroradiology 15: 225-237

Willinsky R, Lasjaunias P, Terbrugger KN et al. (1990) Multiple cerebral arteriovenous malformations. Review of our experience from 203 patients with cerebral vascular lesions. Neuroradiology 32: 207-210

Yasargil MG (1987a) AVMs of the brain, history, embryology, pathological considerations, haemodynamcis, diagnostic studies, microsurgical anatomy, Vol 3A. Thieme, Stuttgart, Germany 7-138 AJNR 15: 1601-1605

Yasargil MG (1987b) Summary of operative results. In: Yasargil MG & McLeod (eds) Micro-neurosurgery, AVM of the brain, clinical non operated cases, cavernous and venous angiomas, neuro-anaesthesia, Vol 3b. Thieme, Stuttgart, pp 250–283

Yeh H, Tew JM, Gartner M (1993) Seizure control after surgery on cerebral arteriovenous malformations. J Neurosurg 78: 12–18

Chapter 6

The Endovascular Treatment of Spinal Vascular Abnormalities

Brian E. Kendall

Introduction

The cardinal principle of embolisation of spinal vascular abnormalities is to reduce or ablate abnormal circulation while preserving the blood supply to the central nervous system.

Anatomy

The arterial blood supply to the spinal cord through an incompletely anastomosing series of longitudinal arteries, described collectively as the anterior and posterolateral spinal arteries. These arteries are joined by a perimedullary arterial network. From this network intramedullary arteries penetrate to supply the parenchyma. The longest vessels, the sulcocommissural arteries penetrate from the anterior spinal artery to supply the grey matter and central white matter. The distributions of these vessels overlap and there is limited anastomosis, with the potential of collateral circulation, between them over short distances.

The peripheral white matter is supplied by smaller end arteries penetrating from the perimedullary network. There is limited overlap between the anterior and peripheral networks which is greater within the cervical and lumbar enlargements.

The posterolateral channels are supplied at many levels by radicular arteries. The supply into the anterior spinal artery is through a more limited number of feeding vessels (radiculomedullary arteries), which are best considered regionally.

1. The upper half of the cervical spinal cord is supplied by the anterior spinal branches arising from the intracranial segments of the vertebral arteries. These spinal arteries usually unite in the region of the foramen magnum but can remain separate. The main flow to the intracranial vertebral artery is from the cervical segments of the same vessels which usually arise from the subclavian arteries. There is variable anastomotic component between the occipital, the deep and the ascending cervical arteries to the vertebral arteries in the suboccipital region through which embolic material can potentially enter the vertebral circulation.

2. The cervicodorsal region is supplied by two to four anterior radiculomedullary arteries originating from the vertebral arteries and/or the costocervical trunks, usually via the deep cervical arteries. Rarely, there is an important supply from the ascending cervical artery.

3. The mid-dorsal spinal cord between D3 and D8 is usually supplied by a single anterior radiculomedullary artery arising from any one of the adjacent intercostal arteries.

4. The lower dorsal and lumbar segments of the spinal cord are predominantly supplied by a single large anterior radiculomedullary artery (arterio radicularis magna of Adamkiewicz). The most frequent origin of this vessel (75%) is from one of the 9th to 12th dorsal segmental arteries but it is important to note that an anterior radiculomedullary artery may arise as high as the fifth dorsal segment or from a lumbar or even a sacral artery. Any of the radicular arteries arising from the lumbar or sacral vessels to supply the lumbar and sacral nerve roots or ascending along the filum terminale may reach the conus and join in a cruciate anastomosis around the spinal cord near the conus medullaris.

Although each of these anastomoses is an alternative route of blood supply to the spinal circulation, equally they are a potential route through which emboli may enter the spinal cord circulation.

In all cases, as a prelude to endovascular treatment of spinal lesions, the blood supply to the neural axis in the region of interest must be clearly defined and any communication between the vessels to be embolised and the spinal circulation must be excluded.

In the cervical region temporary or permanent occlusion of a vertebral artery or an anastomosing external carotid branch after appropriate testing may allow a more complete embolisation to be performed.

The venous drainage of the spinal cord is into longitudinal veins, the most prominent and developed of which are the anterior and posterior spinal veins, which empty into multiple anterior and posterior radicular veins. These are about equal in number, the posterior being of larger calibre. There is free communication with the veins of the posterior fossa above and the lumbar and sacral veins below.

The anterior median spinal vein runs in the anterior median fissure deep to the artery. It is the dominant vein of the lumbar enlargement and it continues along the filum terminale to communicate with the coccygeal and/or sacral plexuses.

The posterior vein(s) are dominant in the dorsal and cervical regions and are particularly large in the dorsal region where they may be tortuous, redundant and somewhat irregular in calibre.

The longitudinal veins are connected by transverse encircling veins the whole forming the perimedullary venous plexus and also by large transmedullary anastomoses running from the anterior to the posterior or posterolateral veins. These anastomoses allow free flow of blood between the anteriorly or posteriorly situated longitudinal veins.

The intrinsic venous drainage of the spinal cord is through radially arranged long and short medullary veins. The former drain the central grey and white matter and receive some short veins from the white matter. The latter drain white matter alone. Both remain mainly horizontally oriented individual vessels as far as the surface of the cord before joining the mainly longitudinal superficial venous system.

In the lumbosacral region the radial system of veins tends to drain mainly towards the anterior median vein; in the thoracic region the drainage tends to be mainly towards the posterior median vein.

Flow can occur freely in all directions in the superficial or perimedullary venous plexus and from it into the posterior fossa. There is also potential for bidirectional flow between the cervical internal and external venous plexuses. In the dorsal and lumbar regions flow occurs normally in an outward direction from the internal plexus through radicular veins. No reflux of blood occurs from the thoracic abdominal or pelvic veins via the external venous plexus through radicular veins into the internal venous plexus. The valvular mechanism appears to be narrowing of the radicular vein plus angulation as it transgresses the dura. The precise working of the mechanism is uncertain but closure may be mediated by increase in the intrathoracic or abdominal pressure.

Embolisation

Embolisation may be an appropriate pre-operative measure to facilitate surgery on hypervascular benign or malignant tumours involving the vertebrae, the meninges, or less commonly, the parenchyma of the spinal cord itself. Such embolic procedures may precede surgery, which by limiting blood loss may allow safer, more definitive or more extensive excision or increase the safety of a biopsy.

Embolisation may also be used as a palliative procedure to reduce pain or arrest haemorrhage. Embolisation with radioactive particles or with ethyl alcohol may be used to delay tumour growth or cause tumour necrosis. Endotumoral injection of acrylics may be used to prevent vertebral collapse.

Spinal Vascular Anomalies

Spinal vascular anomalies may involve:

1. vertebrae
2. epidural tissues
3. the dura
4. the pia
5. the spinal cord parenchyma.

Haemangiomas of the vertebrae are very common occurring in about 11% of the population at autopsy, and they are usually asymptomatic. They may occur at any level but are commonest in the thoracic region.

Pain, neural compression and progressive myelopathy may occur and require treatment. The lesion is uncommonly complicated by compression fracture. The diagnosis is usually evident on plain X-ray which shows a typical honeycomb pattern. In symptomatic lesions expansion of the vertebral body and involvement of the neural arch is common and there may be evidence of epidural extension with spinal cord compression. MRI typically shows a mottled increase in intensity on both T1 and T2 weighted sequences which may be mingled with regions of decreased signal on the T2 weighted sequences.

Selective angiography of the segmental vessels supplying the affected vertebra will usually fill heterogeneous patchy circulation within the haemangiomatous vertebra with extension into paravertebral soft tissue components. The circulation generally persists through the venous phase. Arteriovenous shunting is unusual.

Not all haemangiomas are hypervascular on angiography but those that are symptomatic with increased circulation should be treated with particulate embolisation prior to decompressive laminectomy. Without embolisation decompressive surgery could result in life-threatening haemorrhage.

In the absence of compressive symptoms, embolisation may be helpful for pain relief.

Aneurysmal Bone Cyst

An aneurysmal bone cyst is an expanded cystic space within a bone, sometimes within a pathological region affected by fibrous dysplasia, osteoblastoma or chondrosarcoma. The space is filled with venous blood under tension and surrounded by a thin sclerotic bony rim. Angiography may reveal irregular dilated and tortuous feeding arteries and delayed venous drainage with layering of contrast medium within the cysts. Embolisation may limit access of circulation to the cyst and initiate thrombosis.

Spinal Dural Arteriovenous Fistulas (SDAVF)

SDAVF are the commonest spinal arteriovenous fistulas occurring in middle age and elderly subjects and they have a marked male preponderance (85%) (Kendall & Logue, 1977).

In 1972 Manelfe et al. described a normal vascular structure which is present between two layers in the dura. It consists of a tortuous complex of two or more arterioles leading to a single vein draining to the spinal perimedullary venous plexus. The function of these "glomeruli" is uncertain but may be related to maintenance of more constant blood flow in the spinal veins by regulating inflow to modify the variations in outflow from the perimedullary plexus into the epidural plexus caused by alterations of pressure in the thoracic and abdominal cavities which is transmitted to the enclosed venous systems and hence to the epidural veins.

These glomeruli have a structure similar to dural arteriovenous fistulas draining to the medullary venous plexus and it is possible that the pathophysiology of dural fistulas is due to malfunction of these structures.

In normal circumstances when the spinal cord circulation is outlined during angiography, the venous circulation of the spinal cord drains from the perimedullary to the epidural venous plexuses.

In patients being investigated for symptomatic dural fistulas draining to the perimedullary plexus, injection through the vessels supplying the anterior spinal artery does not outline the perimedullary venous plexus. The venous drainage from the fistula into the perimedullary venous plexus ascends towards the intracranial or descends towards the sacral plexus and does not outline the epidural plexus in the region of the fistula.

It appears, therefore, that two factors are necessary for a dural fistula to become symptomatic: (i) the formation of the fistula itself; and (ii) a restriction of the normal drainage of the veins of the perimedullary venous plexus towards the epidural veins.

Rarely, a dural arteriovenous shunt drains into the epidural venous plexus alone and presents with spinal or root pain or with epidural haemorrhage.

When arterial shunting takes place into the perimedullary plexus, presentation is with a painful myelopathy with mixed motor and sensory impairments. This myelopathy is considered to be due to chronic venous hypertension preventing normal drainage of blood from the spinal cord circulation. The reduction in the arteriovenous pressure gradient in spinal cord tissue results in decreased tissue perfusion and hypoxia of the spinal cord causing dysfunction and eventually to ischaemic changes leading to irreversible necrosis (Aminoff et al., 1974).

The "glomerular"-like structures occur in the dorsal and lumbar dura but not in the cervical dura, a distribution which corresponds with that of dural arteriovenous fistulas.

Paresis, often associated with pain in the back and or lower limbs, generally slowly progressive, but sometimes stepwise with partial remissions, is a usual presenting symptom. Disturbance of bladder and bowel and impotence and sensory disturbance are frequent (Djindian, 1978).

Diagnosis is by magnetic resonance imaging. The enlarged perimedullary veins can generally be shown using T2 weighted fast spinecho imaging, augmented if necessary by gadolinium enhanced dynamic scanning which may also give a clear indication of the site of the shunt.

Myelomalacia affecting the lower dorsal and lumbar cord in a middle aged or elderly male should suggest the diagnosis and encourage search for dilated veins which may not always be conspicuous.

Spinal angiography is necessary as pre-operative procedure. The fistula is generally below D3 level and is usually fed by one, but occasionally by two or three segmental vessels and drained by a single vein into the perimedullary venous plexus. (Merland et al., 1980). The approximate position of the shunt may be suggested by dynamic MRI or even by showing the configuration of a vein leading from it to the plexus. Once the fistula is found it is generally adequate to inject the contralateral artery at the same level and the next three arteries above and below on both sides.

A fistula is not excluded until every artery potentially supplying the dura has been examined adequately. The index of adequacy at each level injected is the production of a capillary blush in the hemivertebra supplied by the selected artery.

If no fistula is found in the spinal canal, consideration should be given to the possibility of an intracranial arteriovenous shunt draining into the spinal perimedullary plexus: this is a rare cause of congestive myelopathy.

The blood supply to the spinal cord in the region of the fistula must be demonstrated and any connection between the vessels supplying the fistula and those supplying the spinal cord must be excluded prior to an embolisation procedure.

If a suitable fistula is localised, the vessel supplying it is catheterised superselectively into the branch leading to the fistula using a microcatheter. Further angiography is performed to confirm the selectivity and exclude neural supply at this site before the fistula is embolised using a small quantity of a 50% mixture of N-butyl cyanoacrylate and lipoidal ultra fluid. This should occlude the fistula plus the first 1-2 cm of the connecting vein.

Isolation of dural fistulas is very simple, by neurosurgical treatment consisting of division of the vein connecting the fistula to the perimedullary plexus with or without destruction of the fistula. (Symon et al., 1984). If there is any doubt regarding suitability of the lesion for embolisation or if there is any technical difficulty in its performance, the fistula should be referred for surgery.

The fistula is composed of very narrow tortuous vessels which are not amenable to particulate embolisation. This procedure will generally produce temporary improvement in symptoms by occlusion of feeding arteries proximal to the fistula. Relapse will occur in over 50% of cases. Particulate embolisation is therefore positively contra indicated in a condition which is permanently cured by liquid embolisation agents or by neurosurgery.

Occlusion of the slow-flow fistula leads to stasis in the dilated venous plexus which may precipitate thrombosis. Following occlusion consideration should be given to low-dose heparin to prevent thrombosis in the distended veins.

Most patients improve after closure of the fistula, but in some the neurological symptoms are only arrested. If improvement does not occur or if there is a relapse of symptoms reinvestigation to show either reopening of the fistula or a second arteriovenous communication should be performed.

Arteriovenous Malformations (AVMs) of the Spinal Cord

AVMs appear to be developmental malformations and are, thus, distinct from the dural fistulas which are acquired malfunctions of developmentally normal structures.

The blood supply to the spinal cord arteriovenous malformations is almost exclusively through anterior and posterior radiculomedullary and radiculopial arteries; very occasionally a small dural supply is demonstrated.

They may occur at any level from the foramen magnum down to the tip of the filum terminale and they may be on the surface of the cord being largely limited to the pia, within the parenchyma or in both situations. They are usually composed of a nidus of abnormal vessels, but they may contain direct fistulas which usually lie superficially within the nidus. A direct fistula, usually on the surface of the cord may also occur without evidence of a nidus.

These lesions differ in other ways from dural AV fistulas. They tend to be high-flow lesions whereas the dural fistulas are slow-flow, and both arterial aneurysms on the supplying vessels and venous aneurysms and ectasias may complicate the lesions. These aneurysms should be sought specifically at the time of pretheraputic angiography since they may be the source of intramedullary or subarachnoid haemorrhage. Rupture of an aneurysm may require emergency treatment by coil embolisation but some unruptured aneurysms regress spontaneously after treatment of an angiomatous malformation.

The arterial supply to a spinal cord AVM is diagnosed using superselective angiography. Because of the disturbed haemodynamics in high-flow fistulas blood may be shunted from adjacent vessels into the vessels supplying the angiomatous malformation/fistula. When the AVM/fistula is treated through the primary supplying vessels such "collateral" circulation will regress spontaneously. Since these vessels also supply the spinal parenchyma they should not be subjected to embolisation.

Angiomatous malformations of the spinal cord (Rosenblum et al., 1980) tend to present much earlier in life than dural arteriovenous fistulas. Symptoms are present in childhood in about 50% of cases and the average age of presentation is in the third decade.

Spinal haemorrhage is the predominant feature in about half of patients and it may be an acute painful paraplegia due to haematomyelia or back pain and sciatica, with or without meningism and confusion, due to spinal subarachnoid haemorrhage, with or without extension into the intracranial cavity.

Haemorrhage tends to recur within a month in 10% and within a year in 40% of cases and it is the cause of death in up to 30% of spinal AVMs. Subdural and epidural haemorrhage are uncommon.

Pain in the back or of segmental distribution is the presenting feature in about 20%. Weakness, sensory change, impotence and bowel and bladder disturbance may all be presenting features and eventually one or more of these symptoms will occur in about 90% of patients. The mechanism of the progressive neurology is less constant than in dural AV fistulas, but shunting into the perimedullary venous plexus is common feature of both groups and venous hypertension with secondary spinal cord hypoxia is one aetiological factor in cases presenting with a progressive myelopathy: steal from the parenchyma through the shunt and compression of neural tissue by distended vessels may also be significant.

The diagnosis is made by MRI. The high-flow angiomatous malformation will generally be evident from the flow voids in large supplying arteries, within the nidus or fistula and in draining veins.

The nidus may expand the spinal cord and be associated with adjacent myelomalcia. In cases presenting with intramedullary or subarachnoid haemorrhage recent blood clot will give typical signal return.

Pretheraputic investigation requires superselective spinal angiography which should be performed as an emergency procedure in cases where haemorrhage is the presenting feature. Although the lesions are within the spinal cord, the vessels concerned within the nidus or fistula do not supply cord substance and many of the lesions are amenable to superselective embolisation through microcatheters introduced into the vessels supplying the lesion, which can then embolised using N-butyl-cyanoacrylate. The embolisation procedure does carry a risk of increasing neurological disability which is difficult to quantify in the individual case but overall is in the region of 5–10%. Since this includes increase in paraparesis, it may be unacceptable in patients presenting with slowly progressive neurology.

For lesions of the filum terminale the morbidity of embolisation is much less and such lesions should be treated early to avoid progression of neurology. The morbidity of surgery for spinal cord AVMs is higher than that of embolisation, apart from those involving the filum terminale which are amenable to either treatment. Surgery is, however, indicated for relief of spinal cord compression by haematoma or thrombosed varices.

References

Aminoff MJ, Barnard RO, Logue V (1974) The pathophysiology of spinal vascular malformations. J Neurol Sci 23: 255–263

Djindjian R (1978) Clinical symptomatology and natural history of arteriovenous malformations of the spinal cord – a study of the clinical aspects and prognosis, based on 150 cases. In: Pia HW, Djindjian R (eds) Spinal angiomas: advanced in diagnosis and therapy. Springer, Berlin, Heidelberg, New York.

Kendall BE, Logue L (1977) Spinal epidural angiomatous malformation draining into intrathecal veins. Neuroradiology 13: 181–189.

Manelfe C, Lazorthes G, Roulleau J (1972) Arteres de la dure-mére rachidiénne chez l'homme. Acta Radiol 13: 829–841

Merland JJ, Riche MC, Chiras J (1980) Intraspinal extramedullary arteriovenous fistulae draining into the medullary veins. J Neuroradiol 7: 221–230

Rosenblum B, Oldfield EH, Doppman JL, di Chiro G (1987) Spinal arteriovenous malformations: a comparison of dural arteriovenous fistulas and intradural AVM's in 81 patients. J Neurosurg 67: 795–802
Symon L, Kuyama H, Kendall B (1984) Dural arteriovenous malformations of the spine: clinical features and surgical results in 55 cases. J Neurosurg 60: 238–247

Chapter 7

The Endovascular Treatment of Carotid and Vertebral Artery Atherosclerotic Disease

Andrew Clifton and Martin M. Brown

The treatment of arterial stenosis by endovascular techniques has the attraction of avoiding open surgery and general anaesthesia which are required for endarterectomy or bypass surgery. Percutaneous transluminal angioplasty (PTA) is frequently performed and is often the first line procedure for stenosis of the peripheral and coronary vessel. There has been reluctance to recommend PTA for the cerebral circulation because of the anxiety about the risks of cerebral embolism (Health and Public Policy Committee, 1983). However, evidence is accumulating that the risks of PTA in the proximal internal carotid and vertebral arteries are no greater than those of PTA at other sites and are similar to the risks of carotid surgery. Clinical trials are now underway assess the procedure and to compare it with carotid endarterectomy, in particular the Carotid Vertebral Artery Transluminal Angioplasty Study. It is possible that if these confirm the safety and efficacy of cerebral vascular PTA, the procedure will become the preferred alternative to surgery in suitable patients. Cerebral vascular PTA also provides a valuable option in experienced centres for the treatment of patients with surgically inaccessible vertebral carotid artery stenosis or for patients who are not fit for surgery.

Disadvantages of Surgery

The benefits of carotid endarterectomy in preventing ipsilateral stroke in recently symptomatic patients with severe internal carotid stenosis has now been convincingly established by the European Carotid Surgery Trial (ECST) (European Carotid Surgery Trialists Collaboration Group, 1991) and the North American Symptomatic Carotid Endarterectomy Trial (NASCET) (North American Symptomatic Carotid Endarterectomy Trial Collaborators, 1991). However, in both trials, there was a significant morbidity and morality associated with surgery and the combined stroke and death rate within 30 days of surgery was 7.5% in the ECST and 5.8% in the NASCET. This combined stroke and death rate is usually the only number that is quoted.

Other important risks include myocardial infarction and pulmonary embolism (Sundt et al., 1975; Rothwell, 1995). Other complications include side effects of anaesthesia, discomfort of intubation, and the risks of pneumonia and of deep vein thrombosis. There is also morbidity and discomfort from the incision. Haematoma in the neck may require exploration. Disability may be caused by damage to the cranial nerves in the neck, most frequently the hypoglossal nerve, resulting in ipsilateral weakness of the tongue. Keloid scar formation may be seen in some patients. One of these minor complications affects at least 10% of patients after carotid endarterectomy. Patients often require a stay in hospital of up to a week and are rarely able to return to full activities for a month. Some patients are not suitable for surgery, such as those with severe ischaemic heart disease, recent myocardial infarction and uncontrolled hypertension. Certain stenoses are not easily accessible by surgery, including those beyond the carotid bifurcation, distal vertebral stenosis and intracranial stenosis.

Advantages of PTA

PTA is performed under local anaesthesia, avoiding the major complications of general anaesthesia and the discomfort and local complications of an incision in the neck. Apart from transient pain in the neck on dilatation of the balloon, discomforts of successful angioplasty are no more than those associated with routine angiography.

The patient need only stay in hospital after PTA for the duration of intravenous Heparin therapy, usually 24–48 hours, and can resume normal activities immediately.

PTA consumes less financial and hospital resources than surgery, only requiring the use of an angiography suite for an hour, and rarely needing admission to an Intensive Treatment Unit. The initial costs are, therefore, much less than surgery (Lambert, 1995).

Mechanisms of PTA

Experimental studies, mainly carried out on animal models, have shown that balloon inflation denudes the endothelium, splits and cracks the atheromatous plaque so that it dehisces from the underlying media, and stretches the media and adventitia (Crawley et al., 1997). Splitting of the atheromatous plaque appears to be essential for successful angioplasty and is the only way that concentric plaque can be dilated. Compression or redistribution of atheromatous material does not occur and dilatation is achieved by increasing the diameter of the whole vessel, hence moving the walls outwards (Castaneda-Zuniga et al., 1980).

After successful angioplasty, a process of repair and remodelling of the artery occurs. This continues throughout the first weeks and possibly months, and the final arterial lumen may become much wider than is apparent immediately after angioplasty. The arterial wall injury caused by angioplasty results in the stimulation of fibroblasts and smooth muscle cells which may be responsible for the remodelling process but may also result in restenosis (Crawley et al., 1997). The factors involving the extent of this reaction are unknown but improvement in luminal diameter with time may be related to replacement of proliferative intima and smooth muscle cells by fibrosis.

Technique of Cerebrovascular PTA

Cerebrovascular PTA is best carried out by an experienced interventional neuroradiologist. The technique consists of percutaneous insertion under local anaesthesia of a sheath into the femoral artery in the groin. Sedation is optional. If access through the femoral artery is difficult, a brachial route may be attempted. This is particularly useful for vertebral PTA. A standard diagnostic catheter is placed in the common carotid artery or the subclavian artery.

Angiograms in multiple projections are then taken of the stenosis and the optimal projection for passage of the guide wire through the stenosis selected. A roadmap is then acquired and after full heparinisation of the patient, usually 5000 u i.v. a guide wire is passed through the stenosis.

The diagnostic catheter is then passed through the stenosis and the guide wire removed. An injection of contrast confirms that the catheter is intraluminal. An exchange wire is then placed through the diagnostic catheter, the diagnostic catheter removed, and an inflatable balloon angioplasty catheter is then passed over the guide wire and maneuvered to straddle the stenosis. The use of radio-opaque markers taped to the neck may aid accurate placement of the balloon angioplasty catheter. The diameter of the balloon is chosen to match the estimated diameter of the vessel with the aim of avoiding overdilatation, usually a 5–6 mm diameter × 4 cm long balloon for lesions at the carotid bifurcation. The ideal balloon catheter has a low-profile tip and a rapid deflation time.

Prior to inflation of the balloon, one ampoule of atropine is given i.v. in order to prevent bradycardia, which may occur from stimulation of the carotid sinus on balloon inflation. The balloon is inflated across the stenosis, up to three times, in order to achieve satisfactory dilatation. Hand-held inflation pressure is usually adequate . Inflation time should be less than 10 seconds. This brief occlusion time limits risk of haemodynamic ischaemia unless the stenosis is so tight that the guide wire occludes the vessel for longer. This is in contrast to carotid endaterectomy where, even if shunts are used, it may take several minutes to insert the shunt after the internal carotid artery has been clamped off. It may be an advantage in some cases to have a second angiography catheter inserted through the opposite femoral artery to allow angiographic views to be taken of the angioplasty result without the need to exchange the balloon catheter for an angiography catheter. This is essential when inserting a stent. After the dilatation, the balloon catheter is withdrawn proximal to the stenosis, and post angioplasty angiograms obtained.

Cerebral Protection Catheters

Theron et al. have advocated the use of cerebral protection catheters (Theron et al., 1990) during cerebrovascular angioplasty, in an attempt to reduce the risks of embolic complications. Their technique involves the use of a triple lumen introducer catheter which is introduced into the common carotid artery. An occlusion balloon catheter is then passed across the stenosis and inflated beyond the stenosis in order to occlude the internal carotid artery. A balloon dilatation catheter is then passed over the occlusive balloon catheter and inflated across the stenosis and withdrawn. The third lumen of the introducer catheter is then used to suck the blood back from below the occluded balloon catheter to remove embolic material. Theron et al. have reported finding cholesterol crystals of up to 200 μm in the aspirate. The technique has the disadvantage of using a large introducer catheter which is difficult to insert and may not be appropriate for very tight stenoses. The complexity of the procedure and particularly the long occlusion time of over ten minutes are likely to increase the hazards. The majority of operators prefer the simplicity of single balloon methods.

Arterial Stents

A stent is a sprung wire mesh which is coiled over a deflated angioplasty balloon and springs open when the balloon is inflated. The stent is then left behind against the wall of the artery upon deflation and withdrawal of the balloon, with the aim of maintaining the patency of the artery (Figure 7.1).

Stents may be particularly useful where there is eccentric calcified plaque as inflation of an angioplasty balloon in this situation often has unsatisfactory results due to recoil of the more normal arterial wall. Stents may also be useful if balloon angioplasty results in dissection with a free flap. It may also be useful and become the treatment of choice for spontaneous carotid dissection (Marks et al., 1994).

Complications of PTA

There are many potential complications of angioplasty. Some degrees of intimal dissection is inevitable, usually localised to the area of plaque. This is the inevitable consequences of successful angioplasty, which involves the splitting of the plaque. However, inadvertent subintimal insertion of the guide wire catheter may result in extensive dissection, leading to vessel occlusion or pseudo-aneurysm formation. Irritation of the wall of the artery by the guide wire or catheter can lead to arterial spasm. This is common, but rarely symptomatic, and resolves spontaneously. Vessel rupture can occur and is recognised in the carotid artery by the sudden onset of severe pain in the neck, associated with extravasation of contrast media out of the vessel. This is a rare complication and in the single case in our series, the extravasation of blood was controlled easily by pressure on the neck. There were no complications other than pain in the neck, and the rupture healed spontaneously without intervention or subsequent sequelae. Angioplasty results in carotid sinus stimulation which frequently leads to bradycardia and rarely leads to brief periods of asystole. The administration of atropine just prior to angioplasty is advised in order to limit this complication. It is essential that the patient is monitored using a standard cardiac monitor during the procedure. Hypotension may occasionally be troublesome for up to 48 hours following the procedure.

Risk factors for symptomatic embolism during PTA have not yet been established but embolism of atheromatous debris or thrombosis during PTA is the main concern. In our experience, risk factors for major stroke after PTA have been a combination of very severe stenosis, a history of angina and "crescendo" transient ischaemic attacks (TIAs). These have also shown to be risk factors for stroke during carotid endarterectomy (Sundt et al., 1975).

Cerebrovascular PTA is, however, tolerated very well by the majority of patients with little discomfort. About half the patients experience brief discomfort in the neck at the site of angioplasty, occasionally radiating to the eye and forehead or scapula (carotidynia). This pain is usually very short lived and only lasts a few seconds during balloon inflation, although it may last up to 48 hours.

Prevention and Management of Complications

All patients scheduled for PTA should be pretreated with antiplatelet agent e.g. aspirin to reduce the chances of embolism during or immediately after PTA and, as mentioned above, full anticoagulation with intravenous heparin 5000 u i.v. prior to

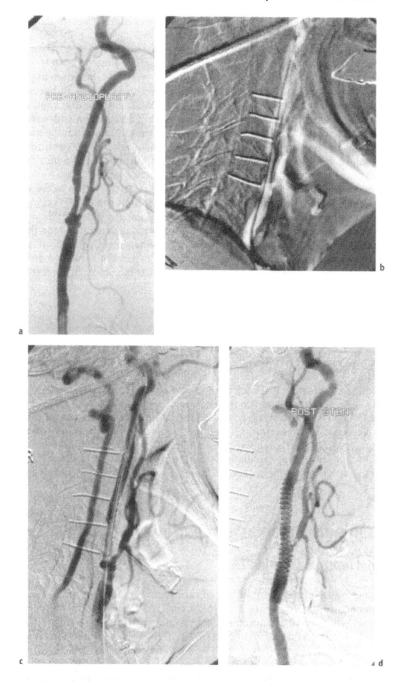

Fig. 7.1. a Digital subtraction angiogram (DSA) showing a long stenosis. Note the eccentric calcification. **b** Digital roadmap showing a graticule in place with the wire across the stenosis. **c** The stent is shown in place across the stenosis, the injection being through a second catheter placed in the brachiocephalic artery. **d** Appearances post stent insertion showing excellent dilatation of the stenosis.

crossing the stenosis and for 24-48 hours after the procedure. The antiplatelet agent should be continued indefinitely afterwards.

The risk of haemodynamic stroke due to temporary occlusion of the treated artery is reduced by limiting the balloon inflation time to a few seconds. Hypotension should be avoided. All patients having carotid bifurcation angioplasty should be pretreated with Atropine to reduce the consequences of baroreceptor stimulation and to prevent bradycardia (Gaines, 1993). This complication is rarely symptomatic and complete asystole very infrequent. If a dissection with a free intraluminal flap is noted during the procedure either from trauma from the guide wire or following balloon inflation, intravenous heparin should be continued after the procedure and the patient anticoagulated with warfarin for 3-6 months. Stent insertion may be appropriate.

One major hazard of PTA is acute occlusion of the artery, either as the result of haemorrhage into the plaque or secondary to dissection. It is much less common for occlusion to occur secondary to thrombus on the damaged intima after successful dilatation. If occlusion does occur, the options for management include thrombolysis, emergency endaterectomy or conservative management with continued anticoagulation. Thrombolysis is unproven and surgery is thought to be more hazardous than conservative management, which is the treatment of choice (Buchan et al., 1988 McCormick et al., 1992).

Monitoring

ECG and frequent blood pressure measurements are mandatory during carotid bifurcation PTA because of the risk of carotid sinus stimulation. A frequent simple neurological examination is useful, such as asking the patient to move all four limbs and to speak. Monitoring of the intracranial artery blood flow with transcranial Doppler (TCD) is useful but it is a research procedure and not mandatory.

After angioplasty, the monitoring requirements are those routinely carried out after angiography, namely regular pulse and blood pressure measurements, examination of the peripheral circulation, and simple neurological observations for 24 hours. Admission to the intensive therapy unit (ITU) is unnecessary in most cases.

Notes About Angioplasty at Various Sites

Proximal Internal Carotid PTA

Indications for carotid PTA are similar to carotid surgery, but at present can only be recommended routinely as part of a clinical trial. PTA should mainly be considered in patients with severe symptomatic stenosis measuring more than 70% linear diameter reduction using ECST or NASCET criteria. Selection of lesions is a matter of experience. The appropriateness of PTA versus surgery for individual patients should be discussed with experienced interventional neuroradiologists and vascular surgeons. The clinical success rate for achieving satisfactory dilatation is over 95% in our centre. Lesions that are rejected are mainly those where a guide wire will not easily pass through the stenosis but would lodge in an ulcer or penetrate the wall because of tortousity of the stenosis. Atheromatous disease of the femoral arteries or iliac vessel is not a drawback. A brachial approach may be possible in some cases. Presence of ulceration visible on ultrasound or angiography is not a contra-indication. These lesions can be treated without complication. The complication rate is thought to be similar to carotid surgery: of a total of 477 cases reported in the literature or at international meetings (Table 7.1), the mean stroke rate at the time of procedure was cumulatively 1.5% for minor or non-disabling stroke and 2.1% for major stroke or death, resulting in an overall rate of 3.6% (Vitek et al., 1986; Burke et al., 1987; Dorros et al., 1990; Insall et al., 1990; Kachel et al., 1991; Millaire et al., 1993; Trinca et al., 1993; Hebrang et al., 1994; Bogey et al., 1994).

The long-term studies to establish the effectiveness of PTA at any site in preventing subsequent stroke are lacking. Randomised clinical trials are, therefore, essential to establish the relative benefits and risks of angioplasty in comparison to surgery and conventional medical treatment. The only randomised medical clinical trial to investigate the risks and benefits of PTA for carotid stenosis in comparison with conventional surgery, the Carotid and Vertebral Artery Transluminal Angioplasty Study (CAVATAS), has just finished. The trial randomised over 500 patients between surgery and angioplasty between 1992 and 1997. The results have been presented at many international meetings. There was no significant difference in the risks of stroke or death related to the procedure between surgery or angioplasty. The rate of any stroke lasting more than 7 days or death within 30 days of first treatment was approximately 10% in both the surgery or endovascular group. Preliminary analysis of long-term survival showed no difference in the rate of ipsilateral stroke or any disabling stroke in patients up to 3 years after randomisation. The full results of the trial are currently being prepared for submission for publication. The rates of stroke and death within thirty days in CAVATAS in both groups are higher than those reported in the literature but not significantly different to ECST (rate of 7.5%). Long-term follow up is not yet available. Hopefully, centres will continue to follow up CAVATAS enrolled patients. Long-term 5 year outcome data for angioplasty patients is scant in the literature. Only when we know how good endovascular treatment is at preventing stroke and death will we truly be able to recommend it. (Ref: Clifton A, on behalf of the CAVATAS collaborators. Preliminary results of the CAVATAS study. Presented at the Working Group on Interventional Neuroradiology, Val d'Isere, January 1998, and British Society of Neuroradiology, Cork, October 1998).

Table 7.1. Risks of carotid PTA

	N	Minor stroke	Major stroke
Bockenheimer & Mathias, 1983	3	0	0
Wiggli & Gratzl, 1983	2	0	0
Tsai et al., 1986	21	0	0
Theron et al., 1987	6	0	0
Freitag et al., 1987	12	0	0
Theron et al., 1990	13	0	0
Kachel et al., 1991	37	0	0
Munari et al., 1992	44	3	1
Eckert et al., 1996	61	2	1
Mathias et al., 1994	166	1	3
Gil-Peralta et al., 1995	62	0	3
Crawley et al., 1998	50	1	2
Total	477	7 (1.5%)	10 (2.1%)

Remodelling

If the immediate result of carotid PTA is suboptimal dilatation of the artery but the plaque can be seen to be fissured by an outline of contrast media, remodelling is likely to result in a good long-term result. For example, in a series of 10 patients with severe carotid stenosis treated by PTA followed by angiography at 12 months, eight showed a significant increase in lumen of up to 40% between the immediate post-PTA results at the site of the treated stenosis and the diameter at 1 year (Crawley et al., 1997) (Figure 7.2). Two patients showed an increase in stenosis, indicating mild restenosis, which was asymptomatic.

Asymptomatic Carotid Stenosis

There is great uncertainty about the benefit of treating asymptomatic patients by carotid endarterectomy because the risks or surgery are higher than the risk of stroke during the first 2 years or so after asymptomatic stenosis is detected. Initial randomised studies did not suggest a significant benefit of surgery, but the most recently published trial reported some benefit in the prevention of any stroke (but not disabling stroke or death) over 5 years (Warlow, 1995; Executive Committee, 1995). It may well be that carotid angioplasty would be safer than surgery in this situation.

Experience of using PTA for distal internal carotid artery stenosis is limited but a few case reports have appeared demonstrating the feasibility of this approach (Brown 1992; Rostmily et al., 1992; Tsai et al., 1992; O'Leary & Clouse, 1994).

Haemodynamic and Embolic Consequences

A significant improvement in cerebral haemodynamics after PTA can be demonstrated by measurement of cerebrovascular reserve, using TCD. In our studies, we have demonstrated an average improvement over 4 weeks after PTA of about 30% in carbon dioxide reactivity in the hemisphere distal to the treated carotid stenosis, implying improved vasodilator capacity secondary to the improvement in perfusion pressure (Markus et al., 1994a)

Monitoring of blood flow in the middle cerebral artery using TCD also allows the detection of emboli during and after the procedure. Monitoring during and after PTA has demonstrated that short duration, high intensity signals are very frequent immediately after PTA and then continue at declining frequency over the next week (Markus et al., 1994). It is likely that many of these are due to platelet aggregation. The emboli detected by TCD after PTA are usually asymptomatic and the duration of the signals suggests that the majority are very small and unlikely to occlude vessels other than the smallest capillaries.

Long-Term Results of Carotid PTA

No adequate long-term follow-up data is available as yet to assess the adequacy of cerebrovascular PTA in the prevention of subsequent stroke. Available data suggests that the majority of carotid lesions in which initial successful dilatation is achieved by PTA remain patent. In larger series, 80–90% of lesions did not show significant restenosis at one year (Munari et al., 1992; Mathias 1994; Eckert et al., 1996).

The Endovascular Treatment of Carotid and Vertebral Artery Atherosclerotic Disease   113

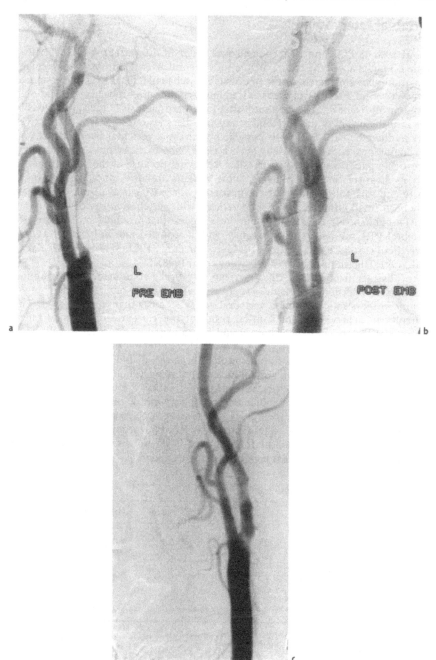

Fig. 7.2. DSA demonstrating remodelling of the arterial wall after percutaneous transluminal balloon angioplasty for very severe internal carotid stenosis at the bifurcation. **a** Immediately pre-angioplasty. **b** Immediately post-angioplasty, showing evidence of residual stenosis and subintimal dissection. **c** One year post-angioplasty with excellent remodelling, resulting in a widely patent lumen.

Vertebral Artery Stenosis

About 10% of TIAs and ischaemic strokes occur in the vertebrobasilar territory. Little is known about the natural history of vertebral artery stenosis. It is reasonable to assume that a recurrence of vertebrobasilar ischaemia distal to a severe stenosis of the vertebral arteries will occur as frequently in the vertebrobasilar circulation as in the carotid. One of the commonest sites for atherosclerosis in the vertebrobasilar tree is at the origin of the vertebral artery and these lesions appear to be relatively easy to dilate by PTA. Surgery is possible on proximal vertebral artery stenosis but is a major procedure. There has been a reluctance to carry out angiography to investigate patients with vertebrobasilar ischaemia because of the perception that only medical treatment is available. Some patients are ideal candidates for angioplasty and this policy should be reconsidered where PTA is available. There have only been small numbers of series of patients with vertebral artery disease treated by PTA published in the literature but these suggest that proximal and mid-portion vertebral PTA can be carried out safely, with a reported morbidity which is even lower than carotid PTA (Table 7.2) (Motarjeme et al., 1982; Mathias, 1987; Kachel et al., 1991; Higashida et al., 1993; Crawley et al., 1998).

An abstract from the North American Cerebral Percutaneous Transluminal Angioplasty Register investigators (Ferguson et al., 1995) reports a lower angiographic success rate in dilating vertebral artery stenosis than at other sites. This difficulty in achieving a good initial result at the vertebral origin may reflect anatomical factors similar to those found at the origin of the renal vessels. Their results parallel our own small series of four, where after excellent initial dilatation in all four subjects with no complications, three out of four showed significant restenosis at one year, though remaining asymptomatic. (Figure 7.3) It is likely that stenting will become the method of choice for treating these particular stenosis. This is now the treatment of choice at our centre, with three successful vertebral stent insertions.

Angioplasty of the distal vertebra artery is more hazardous (Higashida et al., 1993), probably because small perforating vessels which arise above the origin of the posterior inferior cerebellar artery are easily occluded.

Table 7.2. Risks of vertebral PTA

	N	Minor stroke	Major stroke
Motarjeme et al., 1982	13	0	0
Mathias, 1987	6	0	0
Kachel et al., 1991	15	0	0
Higashida et al., 1993	39	0	3
Crawley et al., 1998	4	0	0
Total	77	0	3 (3.9%)

Basilar Artery Stenosis

This is more hazardous than angioplasty in other major vessels because of the likelihood of occluding the penetrating branches of the basilar artery supplying the brain stem. It has only been attempted in fairly desperate situations, such as a

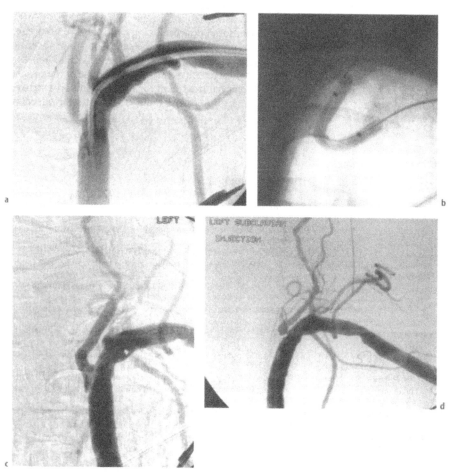

Fig. 7.3. a The injection into the left subclavian artery via the brachial approach shows tight stenosis at the origin of the vertebral artery with post-stenotic dilatation. b The balloon is seen inflated across the stenosis giving excellent dilatation. c Very widely patent lumen post-angioplasty. d One year post-angioplasty, left subclavian injection via femoral route showing marked restenosis.

patient with postural dependent haemodynamic posterior circulation ischaemia associated with severe basilar stenosis. Dramatic success can occur in this situation but the risks are high. Higashida et al. (Higashida et al., 1993) reported two cases of basilar stenosis treated by PTA with good results though a third case treated previously by intra-operative angioplasty by direct vertebral puncture died.

Conclusion

PTA provides an exciting new advance for the treatment of cerebrovascular disease, which may have advantages over surgery or conventional medical treatment.

Appropriate skills in the neurological assessment of patients, interventional neurological assessment of patients, interventional neuroradiology and the application of balloon angioplasty techniques are essential to ensure the safety of the procedure. Randomised trials, such as CAVATAS, are needed to establish the risks and benefits of PTA for cerebrovascular disease. If these confirm the initial promise of the procedure, PTA will become a useful and essential treatment for the prevention of stroke, joining coronary and peripheral PTA as one of the main treatments for vascular disease.

References

Bogey WM, Demasi RJ, Tripp MD, Vithalani R, Johnsrude IS, Powell SC (1994) Percutaneous transluminal angioplasty for subclavian artery stenosis. Am Surg 60: 103-106

Bockenheimer S, Mathias K (1983) Percutaneous transluminal angioplasty in arteriosclerotic internal carotid artery stenosis. AJNR 4: 791-792

Brown MM (1992) Balloon angioplasty for cerebrovascular disease. Neurol Res 14 (supplement): 159-173

Buchan A, Gates P, Pelz D, Barnett HM (1988) Intraluminal thrombus in the cerebral circulation: implications for surgical management. Stroke 19: 681-687

Burke DR, Gordon RL. Mishkin JD, McLean GK, Meranze SG (1987) Percutaneous transluminal angioplasty of subclavian arteries. Radiology 164: 699-704

Castaneda-Zuniga WR, Formanek A, Tadavarthy M et al. (1980) The mechanisms of balloon angioplasty. Radiology 135: 565-571

Crawley F, Clifton A, Markus H, Brown MM (1997) Delayed improvement in carotid artery diameter after carotid angioplasty. Stroke 28(3): 574-579

Crawley F, Brown MM, Clifton AG (1998) Angioplasty and stenting in the carotid and vertebral arteries. Postgrad Med J 74: 7-10

Dorros G, Lewin RF, Jamnadas P, Mathiak LM (1990) Peripheral transluminal angioplasty of the subclavian and innominate arteries utilizing the brachial approach: acute outcome and follow-up. Cathet Cardiovasc Diagn 19: 71-76

Eckert B, Zanella FE, Thie A, Steinmetz J, Zeumer H (1996) Angioplasty of the internal carotid artery: results, complications and follow-up in 61 cases. Cerebrovasc Dis 6: 97-105

European Carotid Surgery Trialists Collaboration Group (1991) MRC European carotid surgery trial: interim results for symptomatic patients with severe (70-99%) or with mild (0-29%) carotid stenosis. Lancet 337: 1235-1243

Executive Committee for the Asymptomatic Carotid Atherosclerosis Study (1995) Endarterectomy for asymptomatic carotid artery stenosis. JAMA 273: 1421-1428

Ferguson RDG, The North American Cerebral Percutaneous Transluminal Angioplasty Register (NACPTAR) investigators (1995) Vascular determinants of successful cerebral percutaneous transluminal angioplasty (CPTA). Neurology 45 (supplement 4): A375 (abstract)

Freitag G, Freitag J, Koch RD (1987) Transluminal angioplasty for the treatment of carotid artery stenosis. Vasa 16: 67-71

Gaines PA (1993) Carotid angioplasty and sinus arrhythmias. Clini Radiol 48: 431-433

Gil-Peralta A, Mayol A, Gonzalez A, et al. (1996) Percutaneous transluminal angioplasty of symptomatic atherosclerotic carotid arteries: results, complications and follow-up. Stroke 27: 2271-2273

Health and Public Policy Committee American College of Physicians (1983) Percutaneous transluminal angioplasty. Ann Int Medi 99: 864-869

Hebrang A, Maskovic J, Tomac B (1994) Percutaneous transluminal angioplasty of the subclavian arteries: long-term results in 52 patients. AJR 156: 1091-1094

Higashida RT, Tsai FY, Halbach V et al. (1993) Transluminal angioplasty for atherosclerotic disease for the vertebral and basilar arteries. J Neurosurg 78: 192-198

Insall RL, Lambert D, Chamberlain J, Proud G, Murthy LN, Loose HW (1990) Percutaneous transluminal angioplasty of the innominate, subclavian and axillary arteries. Eur J Vasc Surg 46: 591-595

Kachel R, Basche ST, Heerklotz I, Grossman K, Endler S (1991) Percutaneous transluminal angioplasty (PTA) of supra-aortic arteries, especially internal carotid artery. Neuroradiology 33: 191-194

Lambert M (1995) Should carotid endarterectomy be purchased? Purchasers need a broader perspective. BMJ 310: 317-318

Marks MP, Dake MD, Steinberg GK, Norbash AM, Lane B (1994) Stent placement for arterial and venous cerebrovascular disease: preliminary experience. Radiology 191: 441-446

Markus HS, Clifton A, Brown MM (1994a) Carotid angioplasty: haemodynamic and embolic consequences. Cerebrovasc Dis 4: 259 (abstract)

Markus HS, Clifton A, Buckenham T, Brown MM (1994b) Carotid angioplasty: detection of embolic signals during and after the procedure. Stroke 25: 2403-2406

Mathias K (1987) Catheter treatment of supra-aortic occlusive vascular disease. Radiologie 27: 547-554

Mathias KD (1994) Percutaneous transluminal angioplasty in supra-aortic artery disease. In: Roubin GS (ed.) Interventional cardiovascular medicine: principles and practice. 256th ed. Churchill Livingstone, New York, pp 745-775

McCormick PM, Spetzler RF, Bailes JE, Zambramski JM, Frey JL (1992) Thrombo-endarterectomy of the symptomatic occluded internal carotid artery. J Neurosurg 76: 752-758

Millaire A, Trinca M, Marache P, de Groote P, Jabinet JL, Ducloux G (1993) Subclavian angioplasty: immediate and late results in 50 patients. Cathet Cardiovasc Diagn 29: 8-17

Motarjeme A, Keifer JW, Zuska AJ (1982) Percutaneous transluminal angioplasty of the brachiocephalic arteries. AJNR 3: 169-174

Munari LM, Belloni G, Perretti A. Gatti A, Moschini L, Porta M (1992) Carotid percutaneous angioplasty. Neurol Res 14 (supplement): 156-158

North American Symptomatic Carotid Endarterectomy Trial Collaborators (1991) Beneficial effect of carotid endarterectomy in symptomatic patients with high-grade carotid stenosis. New Engl J Medi 325: 445-453

O'Leary DH, Clouse ME (1994) Percutaneous transluminal angioplasty of the cavernous carotid artery for recurrent ischaemia. AJNR 5: 644

Rostmily RC, Mayberg MR, Eskridge JM, Goodkin R, Winn HR (1992) Resolution of petrous internal carotid artery stenosis after transluminal angioplasty: case report. J Neurosurg 76: 520-523

Rothwell P (1995) Morbidity and mortality of carotid endarterectomy in the European Carotid Surgery Trial. Cerebrovasc Dis 4: 226 (abstract)

Sundt TM, Sandock BA, Whisnant JP (1975) Carotid endarterectomy: complications and preoperative assessment of risk. Mayo Clin Proc 50: 301-306

Theron J, Courtheoux P, Alachkar F, Bouvard G, Maiza D (1990) New triple coaxial catheter system for carotid angioplasty with cerebral protection. AJNR 11: 869-874

Trinca M, Millaire A, Marache P, Jabinet JL, Sergeant O, Ducloux G (1993) Angioplasty of subclavian arteries. Immediate and mid-term results. Ann Cardiol d'Angeiol (Paris) 42: 127-132

Tsai FY, Matovich V, Hieshima GB et al. (1986)) Percutaneous transluminal angioplasty of the carotid artery. AJNR 7: 349-358

Tsai FY, Higashida R, Meoli C (1992) Percutaneous transluminal angioplasty of extracranial and intracranial arterial stenosis in the head and neck. Intervent Neuroradiol 2: 371-384

Vitek JJ, Keller FS, Duvall ER, Gupta KL, Chandra-Sekar B (1986) Brachiocephalic artery dilation by percutaneous transluminal angioplasty. Radiology 158: 779-785

Warlow CP (1995) Endarterectomy for asymptomatic carotid stenosis? Lancet 345: 1254-1255

Wiggli U, Gratzl O (1983) Transluminal angioplasty of stenotic carotid arteries. Case reports and protocol. Am J Neuroradiol 4: 4793-4795

Chapter 8
Neurological Monitoring During Endovascular Procedures

Steven White and Richard Langford

Introduction

Interventional neuroradiology is relatively safe in most of its applications. However, there is some risk of producing new neurological deficits. These may result from the unintentional occlusion of arterial branches to functional nervous tissue or haemorrhage, either from vessel penetration during the procedure itself or associated with disturbances of regional cerebral haemodynamics.

One large series of embolisation procedures for cerebral arteriovenous malformations (AVMs) had a complication rate of 14% with 1.2% for death or major neurological sequelae (Young & Pile-Spellman, 1994). Cerebral haemorrhage in association with AVM embolisation was seen in 11% of cases in another series, with a poor outcome in 5% (Purdy, et al., 1991).

A range of techniques for monitoring the function of the brain, spinal cord and cranial nerves has been used in an attempt to reduce the risks of endovascular procedures. They are reviewed in this chapter under the following headings:

1. *Provocative pharmacological testing with the superselective injection of drugs (usually sodium amytal or lidocaine).* This has been used particularly during the embolisation of cerebral and spinal AVMs and vascular lesions supplied by the external carotid circulation. Clinical testing for drug-induced neurological changes may be extended by neurophysiological methods (electroencephalography and evoked potentials) before it is considered safe to proceed with embolisation of a particular vessel.

2. *Temporary endovascular occlusion*, commonly using an inflatable balloon, has been applied most frequently to the internal carotid artery. Clinical testing of the ability to tolerate occlusion before permanent sacrifice of the vessel has been supplemented by a number of techniques for assessing cerebrovascular reserve by imaging cerebral blood flow (^{133}xenon static probe, stable xenon-enhanced computed tomography, single photon emission computed tomography and transcranial Doppler ultrasonography), again often with additional neurophysiological monitoring.

3. *Monitoring of AVM haemodynamics using transcranial Doppler ultrasonography, direct measurement of pressure in feeding arteries and monitoring of jugular bulb*

oxygen saturation. These methods have been used to guide the progress of the embolisation procedure. They may also help to identify patients at risk for serious neurological complications, such as brain swelling and haemorrhage, following embolisation or subsequent surgical resections. This can allow early therapeutic intervention to minimise morbidity.

Provocative Pharmacological Testing with Superselective Injection of Drugs

Intracranial Circulation

The technique is based on the Wada test for the lateralisation of language function in candidates for epilepsy surgery (Wada & Rasmussen, 1960), in which sodium amytal is injected through a catheter in the internal carotid artery (ICA) while brief tests of speech and language are performed. The ICA on each side is injected in turn and by observing the clinical effects, cerebral dominance for language can be established with good reliability. The development of microcatheters has led to more selective amytal testing with posterior cerebral artery injections allowing assessment of hippocampal function (Clifford et al., 1988).

Provocative testing with superselective angiography or "superselective anaesthesia functional examination", "SAFE" as it has been called by Young and Pile-Spellman (1994), may be used before the therapeutic embolisation of feeding arteries to AVMs. Each pedicle is studied initially with superselective angiography to look for the presence of normal cerebral branches (Dion & Mathis, 1994). However, small arterial branches supplying normal brain may lie distal to the tip of the microcatheter but not be clearly visualised, with the result that injection of embolic material may produce a deficit in that territory (Barr et al., 1994). A baseline neurological examination is carried out before the provocative test. Sodium amytal mixed with contrast is then injected and an angiogram of the distribution of the drug–contrast mixture obtained. The clinical assessment is repeated, to look for any change in neurological status, focussing on the type of impairment expected from dysfunction in the particular brain region. Gross motor and sensory testing may be inadequate and attention needs to be paid to more subtle changes – for example, when the area of interest involves the dominant parietal lobe or other eloquent cortex whose function is primarily cognitive (Young & Pile-Spellman, 1994). For this reason, the evaluation may be extended with brief neuropsychological testing (Vinuela et al., 1982; Paiva et al., 1995). If an apparently normal arterial branch had been visible on the initial superselective angiogram, a negative SAFE is suspicious. It may indicate that the function of the area of brain it supplies was not adequately screened by the neurological evaluation carried out (Barr et al., 1994).

If the test is negative the branch can be embolised. If the test is positive – a new neurological deficit developing with amytal injection – that particular pedicle is not embolised or the catheter is advanced until SAFE becomes negative. When the test is positive, neurological changes appear rapidly and resolve spontaneously within about 5–10 minutes. If the test is equivocal, it is advisable to repeat it after the initial dose of drug has cleared (Barr et al., 1994).

The decision will sometimes be made to proceed with embolisation, even when SAFE has been positive. If the changes in neurological function are mild, they may be felt to represent an acceptable trade-off to achieve proper treatment of the AVM. A positive SAFE does appear to indicate reliably the deficits which will actually occur if a branch is embolised (Rauch et al., 1992; Han et al., 1994).

Unfortunately, a negative SAFE cannot guarantee that normal brain will not be compromised following embolisation (Dion & Mathis, 1994). A false negative may arise from underinjection of amytal or a sump effect from the high flow to the AVM, the drug by-passing normal brain (Dion & Mathis, 1994; Young & Pile-Spellman, 1994). Fox et al. (1990) have questioned the reliability of SAFE because of the problems with rapid diffusion of amytal through the nidus of the AVM. Subtle neurological changes may also be overlooked in the rather constrained circumstances of testing. Han et al. (1994) describe a patient who developed mild sensory changes in one hand, not recognised as related to the test injection because of discomfort from an intravenous line, who experienced a persistent sensory deficit after embolisation. A deficit may also arise despite a genuinely negative SAFE. Another patient in the same series developed a hemiparesis after embolisation of an AVM, preceded by a negative test. Review of post-embolisation angiograms showed that a normal artery supplying the motor area had apparently been occluded by reflux of the embolic agent (Han et al., 1994). A negative SAFE will not exclude the risk of a range of complications: unanticipated reflux of embolic material into normal vessels, propagation of thrombus after embolisation, direct injury to vessels during catheterisation and brain swelling and haemorrhage arising from haemodynamic changes (Deveikis, 1996).

False positives can result from overinjection of amytal or reflux into normal vessels and generalised sedation from recirculation of amytal may occasionally interfere with testing (Young & Pile-Spellman, 1994).

If the first embolisation has produced incomplete obliteration of the target vessels it may be advisable to repeat SAFE before injecting additional material. Han et al. (1994) had one patient with a negative SAFE, followed by partial embolisation, who developed a transient focal deficit on a second test barbiturate injection. They suggest that this may have arisen from redistribution of blood flow in the AVM and adjacent brain following the first embolisation (Batjer et al., 1989).

Although amytal is the preferred drug for SAFE of intracranial vessels, other barbiturates have been used with apparent safety and reliability. Han et al. (1994) used thiopentone, and methohexitone has been advocated when large or multiple test injections are needed – commonly the case when embolising large AVMs – because of its short half-life and the briefer sedative effects than with amytal (Peters et al., 1993).

Provocative testing of vertebral artery branches can be performed in the same way as for the ICA. However, when injecting branches which may supply the brainstem anaesthetic standby is advisable, since a positive test may precipitate apnoea (Barr et al., 1994).

Dural AVMs may have feeders from multiple intracranial and extracranial sources and can be approached by multistage embolisations with preliminary provocative testing, as for cerebral AVMs (Young & Pile-Spellman, 1994).

SAFE obviously requires the patient to be able to co-operate with testing. If conscious sedation or neuroleptanalgesia is used during interventional neuroradiology, this must be modified to give sufficient alertness for reliable assessment (Young & Pile-Spellman, 1994). However, some groups have carried out embolisation of AVMs under general anaesthesia without any provocative testing at all (Debrun et al., 1997), although this strategy does not command universal agreement (Hopkins & Jenkins, 1997).

External Carotid Territory

Provocative pharmacological testing may be carried out before endovascular procedures involving vessels in the external carotid territory to assess the risks of:

1. Injury to a cranial nerve from compromise of its blood supply (DeVries et al., 1986);
2. Cerebral or brainstem infarction from passage of embolic material through external carotid to internal carotid or vertebral artery anastamoses (Thomas & Walters, 1980).

Horton and Kerber (1986) injected lidocaine into branches of the external carotid artery to test for effects on cranial nerve function prior to the embolisation of facial and dural AVMs and vascular tumours of the head and neck. This seemed to be a reliable technique. However, in one patient with a large glomus tumour, a test injection into a small branch of the right external carotid artery produced no cranial nerve deficit, but did lead to severe vertigo, nystagmus, nausea and vomiting lasting for 30 minutes. This was presumably the result of passage of lidocaine into the posterior circulation. There is clearly some concern about lidocaine being injected into the intracranial circulation because of the risk of seizures or cardiorespiratory arrest (Deveikis, 1996).

To avoid this problem while being confident of testing cranial nerve function adequately, Deveikis (1996) used a two-stage testing protocol. After baseline neurological examination amytal injection was used to test for any evidence of effects on the brain. If this first stage was negative, giving no indication of communication with the intracranial circulation, an injection of lidocaine was given to look for disturbances of cranial nerve function. If both phases were negative the vascular branch was embolised. One patient in whom the middle meningeal artery was catheterised for embolisation of a cavernous dural arteriovenous fistula showed a positive amytal test, developing numbness in the contralateral lower limb, recovering in about 10 minutes. Examination of superselective digital subtraction angiograms showed evidence of collateral flow into the anterior cerebral territory. Several patients had positive lidocaine tests, with the cranial nerve deficits resolving within 5-15 minutes. The fact that initial amytal testing was negative in the patients who developed cranial nerve problems following lidocaine injection, confirmed the view that amytal does not test cranial nerve function.

It is also possible to assess whether branches of the ophthalmic artery can be embolised safely without damaging the retina. Horton and Dawson (1988) gave sequential injections of amytal and lidocaine in a patient with a highly vascular frontal meningioma fed by branches from one ophthalmic artery. Amytal caused no visual deficit but lidocaine produced a scotoma which resolved after 2 minutes, indicating that the retina is sensitive to lidocaine but not amytal.

Spinal Circulation

Spinal AVMs may be amenable to embolisation with superselective catheterisation techniques (Bao & Ling, 1997). Wherever possible, the embolisation should be carried out with the patient awake so that neurological function can be monitored clinically throughout the procedure (Horton et al., 1986). If general anaesthesia is necessary, a wake-up test may be performed to assess neurological status (Young & Pile-Spellman, 1994).

Provocative pharmacological testing is also possible before spinal embolisation. The effects of injections of pentobarbitone and lidocaine into the artery of Adamkiewicz have been examined in a rhesus monkey model (Doppman et al., 1986). Pentobarbitone produced an immediate flaccid paraplegia with the time taken to recover being proportional to the dose and ranging from 10 minutes to more than 1 hour. Lidocaine injection caused an initial brief period of flaccidity which was followed by hyper-reflexia in the lower limbs with fasciculations of the thigh muscles and recovery in 30 minutes. It has been suggested that pentobarbitone acts to suppress activity at synapses and may not be effective for testing spinal cord levels (such as the midthoracic cord) which function mainly as conduction pathways (Doppman et al., 1986; Horton et al., 1986). Lidocaine does block transmission along the major axonal conduction pathways and can be used in combination with pentobarbitone to allow adequate testing (Doppman et al., 1986). A two stage procedure with methohexitone and lidocaine has also been suggested (Barr et al., 1994). However, there would clearly be anxieties about provocative pharmacological testing at the cervical level, because of the risk of producing respiratory compromise.

Test occlusion of spinal AVM feeding vessels with a balloon catheter has also been used to check that there is no change in neurological function before embolisation (Horton et al., 1986).

False positives may occur with spinal provocative testing. Katsuta et al. (1993) describe a patient with a T10 AVM who developed a marked motor and sensory deficit in the lower limbs after lidocaine injection, with a concurrent deterioration in somatosensory evoked potentials (SSEPs). Nevertheless, careful embolisation with a slow fractionated injection of particles was carried out with clinical and SSEP monitoring. Embolisation was stopped when clonus developed on electrical stimulation of the posterior tibial nerve with an upgoing plantar response in one foot. There was some mild deterioration in motor function in the lower limbs after the procedure, but not the gross deficit which the lidocaine test had predicted and sensory function was actually slightly improved. It was suggested that because multiple radicular arteries may connect with the anterior spinal artery, embolisation of one or more may be tolerated, providing flow in the anterior spinal artery is preserved by collaterals. Lidocaine injection was considered to have overestimated the effects of embolisation because the liquid drug had been able to spread quite freely though this vascular network.

Neurophysiological Monitoring in Interventional Neuroradiology: Cerebral AVM Embolisation

Pre-embolisation provocative testing with amytal may be extended by monitoring the electroencephalogram (EEG) to look for changes related to injection of the drug (Rauch et al., 1992; Paiva et al., 1995).

The EEG displays brain electrical activity recorded from scalp electrodes. It can be evaluated systematically in terms of several important characteristics, including: voltage (μV), frequency (in Hz), symmetry or asymmetry and the presence of abnormal waveforms, such as spikes and sharp waves (Binnie et al., 1982; Werner & Kochs, 1995). Conventionally, EEG frequencies are divided into four bands: α (8–13 Hz), β (>13 Hz), θ (4–7 Hz) and δ (less than 4 Hz). Beta frequencies are commonly referred to as "fast activity" and theta and delta frequencies as "slow activity" (with θ sometimes being characterised separately as "intermediate slow activity") (Binnie et al., 1982).

As early as 1937 Gibbs and Lennox had suggested that the EEG might be a practical method for monitoring the depth of anaesthesia (Gibbs et al., 1937). It has subsequently been shown to be very sensitive to the effects of sedative and anaesthetic drugs (Werner & Kochs, 1995). This is the basis for the routine recording of the EEG during the Wada test for language lateralisation in presurgical epilepsy evaluation (Nuwer, 1993). After amytal injection, prominent slow activity rapidly develops in the brain areas which have been perfused by blood carrying the drug, last for anything from 3-10 minutes. The appearance of unilateral EEG slowing limited to the hemisphere ipsilateral to the internal carotid injection indicates that there has been no significant cross-circulation of drug to the opposite hemisphere (in which case bilateral EEG changes will be seen). This helps confirm the validity of the conclusions drawn about language lateralisation from the neuropsychological testing, as well as monitoring the duration of the amytal effect, which varies between patients.

The same principles apply to the application of the EEG during SAFE prior to embolisation procedures (Nuwer, 1993). The EEG is monitored during the superselective amytal injection to see if there is any change. Usually, neither clinical nor EEG changes occur and embolisation may proceed. However, if the EEG does alter sigificantly, this suggests that the vessel injected perfuses functional cortex adjacent to the AVM.

Rauch et al. (1992) used EEG monitoring during SAFE in patients with brain AVMs. They carried out both standard recording and computer generated topographical mapping, which produces colour displays of the distribution of EEG α, β, θ and δ frequency bands. Amytal-related EEG changes were seen as a loss of the normal α activity and an increase in slow activity, loss of α being the more sensitive indicator. On the topographical maps focal changes in EEG activity were apparent as asymmetries. A positive SAFE was defined as the development of either clinical or EEG changes, or both, and occurred in 21% patients. In 11 cases there were EEG changes in the absence of any apparent new neurological deficit on clinical examination. Rauch et al. (1992) felt that EEG changes alone should preclude embolisation, reasoning that they indicate a risk of producing subtle or subclinical changes in neurological function or of reducing the patient's "neurological reserve". This might increase susceptibility to neurological complications following subsequent surgical removal of the AVM. However, although the EEG was in some cases more sensitive than clinical examination, it was clear that both were required. Three patients showed neurological deficits after amytal injection in the absence of any apparent EEG change. It was suggested that this may have been due to action of the amytal on subcortical brain tissue, resulting in little EEG effect. Alternatively, drug action may have been limited to a very localised but functionally significant area of cortex, too small to produce a detectable change in the EEG but able to produce effects which were apparent clinically (Rauch et al. 1992).

The routine baseline EEG is abnormal in many patients with AVMs, commonly showing focal slow activity related to the lesion, sometimes with additional epileptiform features. Paiva et al. (1995) found that these changes are correlated with the size of the AVM nidus and with the Spetzler-Martin index (Spetzler & Martin, 1986). However, they concluded that baseline EEG abnormalities do not prevent new changes being detected quite readily during amytal testing - nor did they have any predicivitive value for problems with the embolisation itself. As in Rauch et al.'s (1992) series, the commonest EEG change seen during a positive test was the appearance or accentuation of focal slow activity. They also found that the EEG was more sensitive (35% positive) than clinical or neuropsychological testing (19% positive).

Drugs used for sedation during interventional neuroradiology may produce EEG changes. Droperidol, for example, has been found to produce more generalised slowing than some other agents and Rauch et al. (1992) recommend avoiding its use during amytal testing. However, in practice, drug-induced global EEG effects will not necessarily prevent the recognition of new focal changes. There is, for example, a large experience in the use of EEG monitoring during carotid endarterectomy to provide warning of impending cerebral ischaemia in patients who are under general anaesthesia, which clearly produces profound modification of the EEG from the waking state (Chemtob & Kearse, 1990; Nuwer, 1993; McGrail, 1996). Indeed, if endovascular procedures are performed in anaesthetised patients (Debrun et al., 1997), amytal testing relying solely upon EEG changes may be the only means of identifying branches supplying functional cortex before embolisation (Dion & Mathis, 1994).

In some centres, EEG monitoring is continued throughout the embolisation procedure, in addition to its use during the preliminary amytal testing (Dion & Mathis, 1994). This is because, as well as being susceptible to drug effects, the EEG is extremely sensitive to cerebral ischaemia and will show immediate changes if regional cerebral blood flow (rCBF) is significantly compromised (McGrail, 1996). If focal EEG changes occur during embolisation itself, this suggests that perfusion of functional brain tissue may have been impaired. This will alert the neuroradiologist to the risk of a neurological deficit. Clearly, if the embolising agent has just been injected into a pedicle, permanent deficits may already have been produced. Nevertheless, the occurrence of EEG changes will raise concerns about further injection in that location. In addition, the suggestion that the EEG is more sensitive than clinical examination (Rauch et al., 1992; Paiva et al., 1995) raises the possibility that a serious neurological deficit may sometimes be avoided if injection of further embolic material is avoided when EEG changes first arise.

The use of an arterial guide wire as an electrode to record the intracranial EEG in several patients with cerebral AVMs prior to embolisation has recently been described and may possibly have clinical application in the future (Nakase et al., 1995).

The EEG represents the background activity of the cerebral cortex. It is possible by the use of averaging techniques to measure sensory evoked potentials - the response of the brain to specific auditory, visual or somatosensory stimulation (Werner & Kochs, 1995). Somatosensory evoked potentials (SSEPs) are sensitive to cerebral ischaemia and have been used for monitoring during carotid procedures (Horsch & Ktenidis, 1996) and aneurysm surgery (Momma et al., 1987). SSEPs represent a further potential method of monitoring for brain ischaemia during interventional neuroradiology, although experience is limited (Dion & Mathis, 1994).

Finally, if complications do occur in association with endovascular procedures. EEG monitoring may have a role in their management as, for example, when barbiturate coma with EEG burst-suppression is induced to attempt to control raised intracranial pressure (Barneti et al., 1987; Verhaegen & Warner, 1995). The EEG may also give some indication of prognosis when a neurological catastrophe has occurred. Paiva et al. (1995) describe one patient who died after developing an intracerebral haematoma, showing an α coma pattern in the EEG while still in the neuroradiology department. This is an EEG pattern, superficially resembling the normal waking α rhythm, but seen in deep coma and often associated with a poor outcome (Westmoreland et al., 1975).

Neurophysiological Monitoring in Interventional Neuroradiology: Spinal AVM Embolisation

Neurophysiological monitoring of spinal cord function with SSEPs during orthopaedic and neurosurgical operations is well established (Gugino & Chabot, 1990; Erwin & Erwin, 1993).

Berenstein et al. (1984) used posterior tibial and median nerve SSEPs for monitoring during embolisation of spinal AVMs and spinal canal tumours. Neuroleptanalgesia with droperidol and fentanyl permitted clinical evaluation of motor function and did not interfere with the recording of the SSEPs. A provocative balloon occlusion test was carried out to assess the potential effects of embolisation with continuous clinical and SSEP assessment. It was considered positive if the peak-to-peak amplitude of the cortical evoked responses or the latency of the early components changed by more than one standard deviation from baseline. SSEPs were felt to represent a reliable indicator of impaired spinal blood flow with neurophysiological changes sometimes preceding the emergence of clinically apparent neurological deficits. SSEPs appeared to be particularly sensitive to any compromise of anterior spinal artery circulation with rapid changes occurring when contrast material was injected into that vessel.

The assumption behind SSEP monitoring is that impending damage to the spinal cord which is severe enough to lead to a motor deficit will also produce SSEP changes. This is appears to be so in most cases but will depend on the nature of the spinal pathology (Gugino & Chabot, 1990). SSEPs reflect dorsal column function and may remain unchanged if a selective injury occurs to the corticospinal tracts (Horton et al., 1986; Lesser et al., 1986). Nevertheless, SSEP monitoring may detect significant cord ischaemia even with anterior spinal artery flow disturbances (Berenstein et al., 1984; Therapeutics and Technology Assessment Subcommittee, 1990).

False positives also occur and many patients with spinal lesions will have abnormal baseline SSEP studies, making satisfactory monitoring during procedures more challenging (Werner & Kochs, 1995).

SSEPs require the averaging of several hundred responses to acquire reproducible waveforms and this takes some minutes, so that real-time feedback is not provided. This may clearly represent a limitation in some monitoring settings, although more advanced signal processing methods may reduce feedback time (John et al., 1988; Gugino & Chabot, 1990).

Motor-evoked potentials can be recorded from peripheral muscles following electrical or magnetic stimulation over the motor cortex or rostral spinal cord and have been used for the direct monitoring of conduction in descending motor pathways during spinal surgery (Edmonds et al., 1989; Zentner, 1989). These methods may be applicable to monitoring during spinal endovascular procedures, but are technically more difficult than SSEP recording and more prone to disturbance from medication effects (Kalkman et al., 1992).

Test Balloon Occlusion of the Carotid Artery

Background

Temporary or permanent carotid occlusion may be considered in a number of situations including: head and neck or skull base tumours; aneurysms which are not readily amenable to surgical clipping; caroticocavernous fistulae and traumatic vascular injuries (Mathis et al., 1994; Young & Pile-Spellman, 1994).

To anticipate the consequences of permanent carotid occlusion a preliminary test occlusion may be carried out. In 1911 Matas used clinical observation of the effect of digital carotid compression to assess tolerance to occlusion of the vessel. However, a range of special investigations is now used to supplement clinical examination in the assessment of cerebrovascular reserve (Mathis et al., 1994). Young and Pile-Spellman (1994) outline one comprehensive protocol. Routine carotid and vertebral angiograms are first performed to assess the integrity of the circle of Willis, with carotid artery compression to evaluate cross filling via the anterior and posterior communicating arteries. A baseline neurological examination is carried out followed by measurement of the velocity of middle cerebral artery (MCA) blood flow by transcranial Doppler ultrasonography (TCD) and of rCBF with stable xenon-enhanced computed tomography (CT). The carotid artery balloon catheter is then inflated and the stump pressure in the carotid artery distal to the balloon recorded. The neurological evaluation is repeated. After some minutes, the xenon rCBF and TCD MCA flow measurements are repeated. Immediately after this a single photon emission computed tomography (SPECT) tracer is injected to enable subsequent imaging of rCBF distribution. This group assess the extent of cerebrovascular reserve further by inducing deliberate hypotension until the patient becomes symptomatic.

Non-tomographic rCBF Measurement With ^{133}Xenon

The intra-arterial clearance method for measuring rCBF with ^{133}xenon (^{133}Xe) has been used for more than 30 years (Anderson, 1996). ^{133}Xe is an inert gas which is a low energy γ emitter and freely diffusible throughout the brain. It may be dissolved in normal saline and injected into the internal carotid artery. The clearance curves are derived from the ^{133}Xe washout measured by collimated external scintillation detectors placed over the head and CBF values in ml/100 g/min are obtained.

Anon et al. (1992) used this technique to measure rCBF during test balloon occlusion in patients with giant intracavernous carotid artery aneurysms. A fall of more than 25–30% from baseline levels in hemispheric or local CBF following inflation of the balloon was regarded as test failure, even if no clinical changes were apparent. An extracranial–intracranial (EC–IC) bypass would then be carried out before permanent carotid occlusion.

A principal limitation of the method is that the computed rCBF values may sometimes not accurately represent areas of low flow because of the "look through" phenomenon (Anderson, 1996). The technique cannot perform fast serial measurements of rCBF, since if the interval between measurements is too short errors may be introduced (Anderson, 1996).

rCBF Measurement With Stable Xenon-Enhanced CT

Stable xenon-enhanced CT provides non-invasive, high resolution, quantitative measurements of rCBF linked to anatomical images (Yonas et al., 1996). A xenon-in-oxygen mixture is inhaled and recent advances have allowed the required xenon concentration to be reduced from 33% to about 28%. This has reduced problems with xenon-induced sensory disturbances and increases in cerebral blood flow which may arise at higher concentrations (Yonas et al., 1996).

Xenon-CT cerebral blood flow mapping has been used to test tolerance to temporary carotid balloon occlusion in patients with skull base tumours or intracranial aneurysms (Steed et al., 1990; Linskey et al., 1994; Witt et al., 1994). Normal CBF is defined as greater than 40 ml/l00 g/min and compromised but adequate CBF as 30–39 ml/100 g/min, with CBF of greater than 30 ml/100 g/min being required to pass the balloon occlusion test (Steed et al., 1990). The emergence of new neurological deficits on test occlusion implies that flow has fallen below the critical threshold for function of 15–23 ml/100 g/min (Jones et al., 1981). Neurological changes do not seem to appear during balloon occlusion until the CBF values in the MCA territory fall to less than 20 ml/100 g/min (Witt et al., 1994). The false negative rate for xenon-CT CBF data during trial balloon occlusion in predicting flow-related infarctions after permanent carotid sacrifice has been estimated at between 3 and 10% (Linskey et al., 1994).

The stable xenon-CT CBF method does have some disadvantages, including the pharmacological effects of the xenon and the need to allow 20 minutes for adequate xenon washout before repeating a study (Yonas et al., 1996). Doubts have also been expressed about the legitimacy of the rCBF values derived from the method (Purdy, 1991).

rCBF Measurement With SPECT

SPECT is now widely used to study rCBF in nuclear medicine with a variety of applications (Mullan et al., 1996). Dynamic SPECT with inhalation of ^{133}Xe was the first method used clinically. It is straighforward, rapid and provides quantitative rCBF values in ml/100 g/min. However, spatial resolution is relatively poor and there are other technical limitations (Mullan et al., 1996).

A number of intravenous agents for static SPECT imaging are now available, the most widely used being ^{99m}Tc-HMPAO (^{99m}Tc-hexamethylpropylamineoxime). This lipophilic tracer rapidly crosses the blood–brain barrier and becomes trapped within cells in a distribution that is proportional to rCBF. The relatively long half-life of ^{99m}Tc-HMPAO (about 6 hours) means that the imaging procedure can be carried out several hours after the agent has been given, but still reflect rCBF at the time of injection. This represents a significant practical advantage over other brain blood-flow methods, particularly in the context of balloon occlusion, since the balloon does not need to be inflated during the scanning process itself but only at the time of the tracer injection.

SPECT imaging has been used quite extensively to assess changes in cerebral perfusion during carotid balloon test occlusion and to assist in the selection of patients likely to be able to tolerate permanent occlusion of the internal carotid artery without developing ischaemic neurological impairment (Monsein et al., 1991; Moody et al., 1991; Peterman et al., 1991; Eckard et al., 1992; Linskey et al., 1994).

Eckard et al. (1992) distinguished three subgroups of patients: (1) those who develop both neurological and rCBF changes during test balloon occlusion; (2) those who do not show any neurological deficit but develop clear rCBF changes; and (3) those who show no neurological deficit and normal or only slightly altered rCBF during trial occlusion. The value of SPECT is in identifying the second group, who cannot safely undergo permanent carotid occlusion, unless EC–IC anastamosis is done first. SPECT may make a major contribution here, since 5–20% patients who show no clinical signs of ischaemia during carotid trial occlusion may still suffer a stroke if permanent occlusion is carried out (Peterman et al., 1991).

Reversible asymmetries of cerebral perfusion demonstrated by SPECT during trial internal carotid balloon occlusion indicate a significant risk for cerebral infarction following permanent occlusion (Peterman et al., 1991; Eckard et al., 1992). Symmetrical rCBF during trial occlusion has been interpreted as suggesting that no new neurological deficit will occur. However, Peterman et al. (1991) emphasize that if peri or postoperative hypotension occurs, critical decreases in cerebral perfusion with deficit may occur despite satisfactory SPECT studies during trial occlusion.

SPECT studies confirm that angiographic evidence of cross-filling from the non-occluded to occluded side is not a good predictor of the ability to tolerate permanent occlusion (Jawad et al., 1977). Significant rCBF changes may develop during trial occlusion even when good angiographic cross-filling has been seen (Peterman et al, 1991).

Unfortunately, the use of SPECT tracers such as ^{99m}Tc-HMPAO does not provide absolute quantitative measurements of rCBF. Semiquantitative ratio values may be obtained if the count-rate for individual areas of interest are expressed as a ratio of the count-rate in a suitable reference area such as the cerebellum, one hemisphere or whole brain. In cerebrovascular disease, the counts in a low flow region might be expressed as a ratio of the counts in the homologous region in the contralateral hemisphere (Moody et al., 1991). However, if blood flow in the reference area cannot be assumed to be normal, the ratio measures may become meaningless (Nakano et al., 1989). Opinion is divided as to whether an adequate internal carotid trial balloon occlusion requires a truly quantitative CBF method, such as xenon-CT (Yonas et al., 1992; Witt et al., 1994). It has been suggested that SPECT may be too sensitive and exclude some patients who could tolerate permanent carotid occlusion without deficit (Yonas et al., 1992; Linskey et al., 1994).

TCD During Trial Carotid Occlusion

TCD provides rapid, non-invasive, quantitative information about blood flow velocity and direction of flow in major intracranial arteries. It is portable and the ability to provide continuous real-time data makes it suitable for monitoring cerebrovascular function in a variety of settings (Taormina & Nichols, 1996).

TCD has been used to assess changes in CBF during carotid trial balloon occlusion (Anon et al., 1991; Young & Pile Spellman, 1994). A reduction in MCA blood flow velocity on the occluded side of more than 25–30% has been considered a test failure. Changes in MCA velocity measured by TCD during manual occlusion of the carotid artery may also have value as a predictor of the clinical and SPECT rCBF response to trial angiographic balloon occlusion (Giller et al., 1993).

TCD monitoring may help in avoiding neurological deficit from thromboembolic complications during balloon occlusion. Valdueza et al. (1994) describe the case of a child with a rhabdomyosarcoma of the neck undergoing internal carotid balloon occlusion. TCD detected thromboembolism in the Ml segment of the ipsilateral MCA with a good result following termination of the procedure and thrombolysis with urokinase.

TCD does, however, have several limitations (Linskey et al., 1994; Taormina & Nichols, 1996). Although it gives flow velocities, it does not measure CBF directly. The flow values themselves are derived only from the major vessels and give little information about more distal blood flow and flow in border-zones. TCD requires an accessible "ultrasound window" in the skull. Anything from 5 to 15% of patients will have inadequate windows, so that no study will be possible or it will be incomplete;

this may be a greater problem in elderly patients (Taormina & Nichols, 1996). The technique is also highly dependent on operator skill to produce reliable results.

Neurophysiological Monitoring During Trial Carotid Occlusion

The extensive experience with EEG monitoring during carotid endarterectomy has confirmed that there is a close relationship between cerebral electrical activity recorded from the scalp and CBF (Sharbrough et al., 1973; McGrail, 1996). The EEG is valuable in monitoring patients during trial balloon occlusion of the carotid artery, since EEG changes may precede clinical signs of cerebral ischaemia (Monsein et al., 1991; Cloughesy et al., 1993; McGrail, 1996). This enables the EEG to contribute to the identification of patients who will be unlikely to tolerate permanent carotid occlusion without developing neurological deficits and who may first need EC–IC anastomosis.

At University of California, Los Angeles (UCLA), continuous EEG monitoring is used during trial carotid occlusions under neuroleptanalgesia (Cloughesy et al., 1993), with a similar procedure to the one for provocative pharmacological testing prior to AVM embolisation (Rauch et al., 1992). A standard EEG is recorded for real-time visual interpretation together with topographical EEG frequency mapping. Paediatric disc electrodes are used on the scalp to record the EEG, since these are quite small and obscure the angiographic image to a lesser degree than standard adult electrodes. The use of needle electrodes will also achieve this, but may be less well tolerated if the patient is awake. The EEG is monitored continuously for the 30 minutes during which the balloon is inflated, together with neurological and cognitive testing to assess the clinical state. The test is aborted if the patient fails at any stage, by either EEG or clinical criteria. EEG failure was defined as an attenuation of alpha activity or an increase in slow activity. If the EEG change was borderline, traditional visual assessment was supplemented by the topographical mapping. It appeared that the emergence of δ slowing was more likely to be a significant predictor of neurological deficit than a selective reducton in α activity. However, there could also be false negatives from EEG monitoring. One patient who had no EEG change developed neurological signs after 3 minutes of carotid balloon occlusion, with ideomotor apraxia, dyscalculia and language disturbance.

SSEPs have been used for intraoperative brain monitoring during carotid surgery (Horsch & Ktenidis, 1996) and might also be applicable to trial balloon occlusion. However, there is concern that while this method may monitor central cortical regions quite effectively, broader hemispheric coverage of the kind given by EEG is needed for adequate assessment of collateral flow during balloon occlusion (Kearse et al., 1992; Cloughesy et al., 1993). Nevertheless, there may be specific situations where evoked potential monitoring could be particularly appropriate. Aymard et al. (1992), for example, suggest that monitoring brainstem auditory evoked potentials might be useful during endovascular procedures on giant basilar aneurysms.

Measurement of AVM Haemodynamics

TCD Monitoring During AVM Embolisation

The effects of AVMs on cerebral haemodynamics have been studied quite extensively (Kader & Young, 1996). These changes are presumed to relate to the low-resistance properties of the AVM, with high blood flow through the lesion and resultant hypoperfusion of surrounding brain tissue (Batjer et al., 1989). Arterial feeders to an AVM are characterised by high flow velocity – which may exceed 900 ml/min (Manchola et al., 1993) – low pulsatility and low perfusion pressure and the cerebrovascular reactivity to carbon dioxide is reduced (Kader & Young, 1996; Lam & Newell, 1996). The changes in haemodynamics following AVM embolisation and resection have also been studied with normalisation of flow velocity, pulsatility and reactivity being reported (Chioffi et al., 1992; Lam & Newell, 1996).

During treatment of AVMs TCD may be useful (1) to detect non-invasively the presence of residual AVM (on the basis of asymmetrical flow velocities) ; and (2) in the diagnosis and management of the hyperfusion syndrome (Lam & Newell, 1996). A serious complication of AVM embolisation or resection is the occurrence of severe brain swelling and haemorrhage. According to the "normal perfusion pressure breakthrough" theory (Spetzler et al., 1978), normal vessels surrounding the AVM lose the capacity for autoregulation when exposed to chronically reduced perfusion pressures, resulting from steal effects from high flow AVMs. After occlusion of the high flow – low resistance AVM, the pressure is restored to normal levels, the vessels cannot respond appropriately and this leads to brain swelling and haemorrhage. This view has been challenged and an alternative theory proposed which is based on occlusive hyperaemia from venous obstruction (Al-Rodhan et al., 1993). However, whatever the precise mechanism, it is clear that the brain swelling and haemorrhage after AVM resection or embolisation are related to an increase in hemispheric perfusion occurring after treatment (Lam & Newell, 1996).

There is a clear relationship between TCD flow velocity measurements after preoperative embolisation and the occurrence of complications following the subsequent surgery. If the main feeder flow velocity remains higher than 120 cm/s after embolisation, the incidence of postoperative cerebral oedema and haemorrhage is significantly higher than when the velocity is less than this value (Chioffi et al., 1993). TCD appears to be a useful non-invasive method of assessing shunt flow in AVMs. It may allow monitoring of haemodynamic changes following embolisation and guide decisions about further stages of embolisation and the timing of subsequent surgery.

TCD monitoring during AVM resection or embolisation may allow the rapid detection of complications, enabling treatment to be initiated at an early stage. Lam and Newell (1996) report one patient who showed an immediate ispilateral increase in MCA flow velocity following resection of a parieto-occipital AVM, associated with sudden brain swelling not responsive to hyperventilation. He was treated with a high-dose propofol infusion. This resulted in equalisation of the MCA flow velocities on the two sides with improvement in the oedema. He was maintained on a propofol infusion for 24 hours and then made an uneventful recovery.

Further technical advances, for example, in laser-Doppler and thermal diffusion flowmetry may facilitate monitoring of this kind (Bolognese et al., 1993; Carter, 1996).

Direct Measurement of Pressure in AVM Feeding Arteries

The pressure in feeding arteries to AVMs can be measured quite simply through the angiographic microcatheters during endovascular procedures (Jungreis et al., 1989). There is evidence that monitoring changes in these pressures may be useful as a guide to the progress of the embolisation, as well as providing warning about which patients are at high risk of developing complications after the procedure.

The arterial feeders supplying AVMs have significantly reduced pressures which rise rapidly when the low-resistance AVM pathway is obliterated during embolisation (Duckwiler et al., 1989; Jungreis & Horton, 1989; Jungreis et al., 1989). Jungreis et al. (1989) observed an average rise in mean arterial pressure of about 27 mmHg in feeders following embolisation. As TCD studies confirm, these pressure changes are inversely related to flow, the flow velocity in the feeding arteries falling as the pressure increases (Chioffi et al., 1993). Pressure changes may be discernible earlier than the visible slowing of flow seen on fluoroscopy (Duckwiler et al., 1989: Jungreis et al., 1989) and appear to be a more sensitive guide to haemodynamic changes and the progress of the embolisation. Jungreis and Horton (1989) found that when feeder pressure had increased after the infusion of polyvinyl alcohol (PVA) particles, further infusion of particulate material would lead to slowing of flow and haemostasis. If pressure did not increase, they changed to a larger-sized particle to continue the embolisation. Similarly, Duckweiler et al. (1989) found serial pressure measurements helpful in understanding the haemodynamic changes during embolisation of a dural AVM and in indicating the need to occlude the distal transverse and sigmoid sinuses.

Pressure measurements may help identify patients at risk of brain swelling and haemorrhage after obliteration of the AVM. If pressures in feeding arteries and draining veins indicate a cerebral perfusion pressure below the limit of the autoregulatory capacity, the risk of complications may be high (Nornes, 1984; Spetzler et al., 1987). Barnett et al. (1987) also identify low feeding artery pressures before AVM excision as a risk factor and adopted a rigorous postoperative neurointensive care regime in such patients. Especially large increases in feeding artery pressure after embolisation may indicate a risk of normal perfusion pressure breakthrough, but the thresholds for pressure tolerance are not yet clearly defined (Duckwiler et al., 1989).

Continuous Monitoring of Jugular Bulb Oxygen Saturation During AVM Embolisation

Internal jugular bulb venous sampling was first described in 1927 (Meyerson et al., 1927). There has been considerable recent interest in the application of fibreoptic jugular bulb venous oximetry in the monitoring of cerebral blood flow and metabolism in neurosurgical intensive care (Werner & Kochs, 1995). The oxygen saturation of the blood draining the cerebral hemispheres provides information about the global metabolic demand of the brain in relation to its oxygen supply (Gunn et al., 1995; Mayberg & Lam, 1996). The normal value for jugular bulb oxygen saturation (S_jO_2) is between about 60 to 75% and values greater than 90% indicate hyperaemia (Mayberg & Lam, 1996).

Katayama et al. (1994) monitored S_jO_2 during preoperative embolisation in patients with large supratentorial AVMs. The S_jO_2 was high and often exceeded the 90% level. There was a positive correlation between the S_jO_2 and the estimated volume of the AVM. Higher S_jO_2 levels apparently reflected a larger shunt flow through the AVM and were associated with evidence of steal. The S_jO_2 decreased progressively during embolisation procedures. The pattern of the fall in S_jO_2 was related to the type of embolic material used. With NBCA (N-butyl-cyanoacrylate) S_jO_2 might only show a small decrease initially, but the decline became more pronounced as embolisation progressed with a large drop after the final infusion of NBCA. However, when polyfilament polyethylene threads or PVA particles were used a more gradual fall in S_jO_2 was seen, as the number of injected threads or particles increased.

The S_jO_2 in patients with AVMs represents a composite of the oxygen saturation of the shunt flow and of the perfusion flow and a shunt flow ratio can be calculated. Katayama et al. (1994) concluded that quantification of the shunt flow ratio has significant clinical implications for the timing of surgery on AVMs, since a large shunt flow appears to be the single most important predictor of postoperative hyperaemic complications (Spetzler et al., 1978). Circulatory breakthrough caused by an abrupt conversion of a large shunt flow to perfusion flow in previously hypoperfused brain tissue with defective auroregulation is suggested as the basis of hyperaemic complications following AVM obliteration (Spetzler et al., 1978). Evaluation of the ratio between shunt flow and perfusion flow may, therefore, be useful in predicting the risk of postoperative brain swelling and haemorrhage. A staged preoperative reduction in the shunt flow will reduce this risk.

Continuous monitoring of S_jO_2 may provide real-time information to help decide when embolisation has progressed sufficiently to reduce the risk of postoperative brain swelling and haemorrhage. There is a high risk of hyperaemic complications when the S_jO_2 is not reduced to below 90% by embolisation (Katayama et al., 1994). Patients with CT evidence of brain swelling after AVM resection had shown a higher S_jO_2 following preoperative embolisation procedures (Katayama et al., 1994).

Conclusion

It is apparent that many methods can be used to monitor neurological function and rCBF during interventional neuroradiology. There is good agreement on the value of particular approaches: for example, the use of provocative functional testing with the superselective injection of amytal and lidocaine. However, in other cases there is diversity of opinion: for example, over the relative merits of particular techniques for measuring rCBF, or the value of SSEP monitoring in identifying ischaemic changes. Other procedures, such as TCD and S_jO_2 monitoring, have been applied in neuroradiology only relatively recently and their role is still being defined. However, it seems clear that as the application of endovascular procedures becomes more widespread and more complex, the capacity to monitor various aspects of central nervous system function will become increasingly important in ensuring a safe outcome.

Summary

Interventional neuroradiology is relatively safe. However, there is some risk of producing neurological deficits, from inadvertent occlusion of arterial branches to functional nervous tissue or from haemorrhage. There have been various approaches to monitoring the function of the brain, cranial nerves and spinal cord during endovascular procedures in an attempt to reduce this risk. A diverse range of methods has been used:

1. *Provocative pharmacological testing with the superselective injection of drugs (usually sodium amytal or lidocaine)* clinical evaluation for drug-induced neurological changes may be supplemented with neurophysiological monitoring (EEG and evoked potentials) to assess the safety of embolizing particular feeding vessels to arteriovenous malformations (AVMs).

2. *Test balloon occlusion of a vessel, most commonly the internal carotid artery* with neurological evaluation, neurophysiological monitoring and measurement of cerebral blood flow (^{133}Xe static probe, stable xenon-enhanced CT, SPECT, TCD) being used to assess cerebrovascular reserve and the patient's ability to tolerate permanent occlusion of that vessel.

3. *Monitoring of arteriovenous malformation haemodynamics with transcranial Doppler ultrasonography, direct measurement of feeding artery pressures or monitoring of jugular bulb oxygen saturation*: to guide the embolisation procedure itself and to identify patients who may be at risk for subsequent neurological complications (brain swelling and haemorrhage), permitting early intervention to reduce morbidity. The current applications of these monitoring techniques in interventional neuroradiology are reviewed and their limitations considered.

References

Al-Rodhan NRF, Sundt TM, Piepgras DG et al. (1993) Occlusive hyperemia: a theory of the hemodynamic complications following resection of intracerebral arteriovenous malformations. J Neurosurg 78: 167–175

Anderson RE (1996) Cerebral blood flow xenon-133. In: Meyer FB (ed.) Cerebral blood flow. Neurosurgery Clinics of North America vol 7, pp 703–708

Anon VV, Aymard A, Gobin YP et al. (1992) Balloon occlusion of the internal carotid artery in 40 cases of giant intracavernous aneurysm: technical aspects, cerebral monitoring and results. Neuroradiology 34: 245–251

Aymard A, Hodes JE, Rufenacht D, Merland JJ (1992) Endovascular treatment of a giant fusiform aneurysm of the entire basilar artery. AJNR 13: 1143–1146

Bao Y-H, Ling F (1997) Classification and therapeutic modalities of spinal vascular malformations in 80 patients. Neurosurgery 40: 75–81

Barnett GH, Little JR, Ebrahim ZY, Jones SC, Friel HT (1987) Cerebral circulation during arteriovenous malformation operation. Neurosurgery 20: 836–842

Barr JD, Mathis JM, Horton JA (1994) Provocative pharmacologic testing during arterial embolization. In: Hopkins LN (ed.) Endovascular approach to central nervous system disease. Neurosurgery Clinics of North America vol 5, pp 403–411

Batjer HH, Purdy PD, Giller CA, Samson DS (1989) Evidence of redistribution of cerebral blood flow during treatment for an intracranial areriovenous malformation. Neurosurgery 25: 599–605

Berenstein A, Young W, Ransohoff J, Benjamin V, Merkin H (1984) Somatosensory evoked potentials during spinal angiography and therapeutic transvascular embolization. J Neurosurg 60: 777–785

Binnie CD, Rowan AJ, Guffer TH (1982) A manual of electroencephalographic technology. Cambridge University Press, Cambridge.

Bolognese P, Miller JI, Heger IM, Milhorat TH (1993) Laser-Doppler flowmetry in neurosurgery. J Neurosurg Anesthesiol 5: 151–158

Carter LP (1996) Thermal diffusion flowmetry. In: Meyer FB (ed.) Cerebral blood flow. Neurosurgery Clinics of North America vol 7, pp 749–754

Chemtob G, Kearse KA (1990) The use of electroencephalography in carotid endarterectomy. Int Anesthesiol Clin 28: 143–146

Chioffi F, Pasqualin A, Beltramello A, Da Pian R (1992) Hemodynamic effects of preoperative embolization in cerebral arteriovenous malformations: evaluation with transcranial Doppler sonography. Neurosurgery 31: 877–885

Clifford JR, Nichols DA, Sharbrough FW et al. (1988) Selective posterior cerebral artery amytal test for evaluation of memory function before surgery for temporal lobe seizure. Radiology 168: 787–793

Cloughesy TF, Nuwer MR, Hoch D et al. (1993) Monitoring carotid test occlusion with continuous EEG and clinical examination. J Clin Neurophysiol 10: 363–369

Debrun GM, Aletich V, Ausman JI, Charbel F, Dujovny M (1997) Embolization of the nidus of brain arteriovenous malformations with *n*-butyl cyanoacrylate. Neurosurgery 40: 112–121

Deveikis JP (1996) Sequential injections of amobarbital sodium and lidocaine for provocative neurologic testing in the external carotid circulation. AJNR 17: 1143–1147

DeVries N, Versluis RJJ, Valk J et al. (1986) Facial nerve paralysis following embolization for severe epistaxis. Laryngol Otol 100: 207-210

Dion JE, Mathis JM (1994) Cranial arteriovenous malformations: the role of embolization and stereotactic surgery. In Hopkins LN (ed.) Endovascular approach to central nervous system disease. Neurosurgery Clinics of North America vol 5, pp 459-474

Doppman JL, Girton RT, Oldfield EH (1986) Spinal Wada test. Radiology 161: 319-321

Duckwiler G, Dion J, Vinuela F et al. (1989) Intravascular microcatheter pressure monitoring: Experimental results and early clinical evaluation. AJNR 11: 169-175

Eckard DA, Purdy PD, Bonte FJ (1992) Temporary balloon occlusion of the carotid artery combined with brain blood flow imaging as a test to predict tolerance prior to permanent carotid sacrifice. AJNR 13: 1565-1569

Edmonds HL, Paloheimo MP, Backman MH et al. (1989) Transcranial magnetic motor evoked potentials (tcMMEP) for functional monitoring of motor pathways during scoliosis surgery. Spine 14: 683-686

Erwin CW, Erwin AC (1993) Up and down the spinal cord: Intraoperative monitoring of sensory and motor pathways. J Clin Neurophysiol 10: 425-436

Fox AJ, Pelz DM, Lee DH (1990) Arteriovenous malformations of the brain: recent results of endovascular therapy. Radiology 177: 51-57

Gibbs FA, Gibbs EL, Lennox WG (1937) Effects on the electro-encephalogram of certain drugs which influence nervous activity. Arch Int Med 60: 154-166

Giller CA, Mathews D, Walker B, Purdy PD, Roseland A (1993) Prediction of tolerance to carotid artery occlusion using transcranial Doppler ultrasound (Abstract). J Neurosurg 78: 366A-367A

Gugino V, Chabot RJ (1990) Somatosensory evoked potentials. Int Anesthesiol Clin 28: 154-164

Gunn HC, Matta BF, Lam AM, Mayberg TS (1995) Accuracy of continuous jugular bulb venous oximetry during intracranial surgery. J Neurosurg Anesthesiol 7: 174-177

Han MH, Chang KH, Han DH et al. (1994) Preembolization functional evaluation in supratentorial cerebral arteriovenous malformations with superselective intraarterial injection of thiopental sodium. Acta Radiol 35: 212-216

Hopkins LN, Jenkins JA (1997) Comment. Neurosurgery 40: 120-121

Horsch S, Ktenidis K (1996) Intraoperative use of somatosensory evoked potentials for brain monitoring during carotid surgery. In: Meyer FB (ed.) Cerebral blood flow. Neurosurgery Clinics of North America vol 7, pp 693-702

Horton JA, Dawson RC (1988) Retinal Wada test. AJNR 9: 1167-1168

Horton JA, Kerber CW (1986) Lidocaine injection into external carotid branches: provocative test to preserve cranial nerve function in therapeutic embolization AJNR 7: 105-108

Horton JA, Latchaw RE, Gold LHA, Pang D (1986) Embolization of intramedullary arteriovenous malformations of the spinal cord. AJNR 7: 113-118

Jawad K, Miller JD, Wyper DJ, Rowan JO (1977) Measurement of CBF and carotid artery pressure compared with cerebral angiography in assessing collateral blood supply after carotid ligation. J Neurosurg 46: 185-196

John ER, Chabot RJ, Pricheps LS et al. (1988) Real-time intraoperative monitoring during neurosurgical and neuroradiological procedures. J Clin Neurophysiol 6: 125-158

Jones TH, Morowetz RB, Crowell RM et al. (1981) Thresholds of focal cerebral ischemia in awake monkeys. J Neurosurg 54: 773-782

Jungreis CA, Horton JA (1989) Pressure changes in the arterial feeder to a cerebral AVM as a guide to monitoring therapeutic embolization. AJNR 10: 1057-1060

Jungreis CA, Horton JA, Hecht ST (1989) Blood pressure changes in feeders to cerebral arteriovenous malformations during therapeutic embolization. AJNR 10: 575-577

Kader A, Young WL (1996) The effects of intracranial arteriovenous malformations on cerebral hemodynamics. In: Meyer FB (ed.) Cerebral blood flow. Neurosurgery Clinics of North America vol 7, 767-781

Kalkman CJ, Drummond JC, Ribberink AA et al. (1992) Effects of propofol, etomidate, midazolam and fentanyl on motor evoked responses to transcranial electrical or magnetic stimulation in humans. Anesthesiology 76: 502- 509

Katayama Y, Tsubokawa T, Hirayama T, Himi K (1994) Continuous monitoring of jugular bulb oxygen saturation as a measure of the shunt flow of cerebral arteriovenous malformations. J Neurosurg 80: 826-833

Katsuta T, Morioka T, Hasuo K et al. (1993) Discrepancy between provocative test and clinical results following endovascular obliteration of spinal arteriovenous malformation. Surg Neurol 40: 142-145

Kearse LA, Brown EN, McPeck K (1992) Somatosensory evoked potentials sensitivity relative to electroencephalography for cerebral ischemia during carotid endarterectomy. Stroke 23: 498-505

Lam AM, Newell DW (1996) Intraoperative use of transcranial doppler ultrasonography. Neurosurgery Clinics of North America vol 7, pp 709-722

Lesser RP, Raudzens P, Luders H et al. (1986) Post-operative neurological deficits may occur despite unchanged intraoperative somatosensory evoked potentials. Ann Neurol 19: 22-25

Linskey ME, Jungreis CA, Yonas H et al. (1994) Stroke risk after abrupt internal carotid artery sacrifice: Accuracy of preoperative assessment with balloon test occlusion and stable xenon-enhanced CT. AJNR 15: 829-843

Manchola IF, De Salles AAF, Foo TK et al. (1993) Arteriovenous malformation hemodynamics: a transcranial Doppler study. Neurosurgery 33: 556-562

Mast H, Mohr JP, Thompson JLP et al. (1995) Transcranial Doppler ultrasonography in cerebral arteriovenous malformations. Diagnostic sensitivity and association of flow velocity with spontaneous hemorrhage and focal neurological deficit. Stroke 26: 1024-1027

Matas R (1911) Testing the efficiency of the collateral circulation as a preliminary to the occlusion of the great surgical arteries. Ann Surg 53: 1-43

Mathis JM, Barr JD, Horton JA (1994) Therapeutic occlusion of major vessels, test occlusion and techniques. In: Hopkins LN (ed.) Endovascular approach to central nervous system disease. Neurosurgery Clinics of North America vol 5, pp 393-401

Mayberg TS, Lam AM (1996) Jugular bulb oximetry for the monitoring of cerebral blood flow and metabolism. In: Meyer FB (ed.) Cerebral blood flow. Neurosurgery Clinics of North America of North America vol 7, pp 755-765

McGrail KM (1996) Intraoperative use of electroencephalography as an assessment of cerebral blood flow. In: Meyer FB (ed.) Cerebral blood flow. Neurosurgery Clinics of North America vol 7, pp 685-692

Meyerson A, Halloran RD, Hirsh HL (1927) Technique for obtaining blood from the internal jugular vein and carotid artery. Arch Neurol Psychiatr 17: 807-809

Momma F, Wang A-D, Symon L (1987) Effects of temporary arterial occlusion on somatosensory evoked responses in aneurysm surgery. Surg Neurol 27: 343-352

Monsein LH, Jeffery PJ, van Heerden BB et al. (1991) Assessing adequacy of collateral circulation during balloon test occlusion of the internal carotid artery with ^{99m}Tc-HMPAO SPECT. AJNR 12: 1045-1051

Moody EB, Dawson RC, Sandier MP (1991) ^{99m}Tc-HMPAO SPECT imaging in interventional neuroradiology: validation of balloon test occlusion. AJNR 12: 1043-1044.

Mullan BP, O'Connor MK, Hung JC (1996) Single photon emission computed tomography brain imaging. In: Meyer FB (ed.) Cerebral blood flow. Neurosurgery Clinics of North America vol 7, pp 617-651

Nakano S, Kinoshita K, Jinnouchi S, Hoshi H, Watanabe K (1989) Critical cerebral blood flow thresholds studied by SPECT using xenon-133 and iodine-123 Iodoamphetamine. J Nucl Med 30: 337-342

Nakase H, Ohnishi H, Touho H et al. (1995) An intra-arterial electrode for intracranial electroencephalogram recordings. Acta Neurochirurg 136: 103-105

Nornes H (1984) Quantitation of altered hemodynamics. In: Wilson CB, Stein BM (eds) Intracranial arteriovenous malformations. Williams & Wilkins, Baltimore, pp 32-43

Nuwer MR (1993) Intraoperative electroencephalography. J Clin Neurophysiol 10: 437-444

Paiva T, Campos J, Baeta E et al. (1995) EEG monitoring during endovascular embolization of cerebral arteriovenous malformations. Electroencephalog Clin Neurophysiol 95: 3-13

Peterman SB, Taylor A, Hoffman JC (1991) Improved detection of cerebral hypoperfusion with internal carotid balloon test occlusion and ^{99m}Tc-HMPAO cerebral perfusion SPECT imaging. AJNR 12: 1035-1041

Peters KR, Quisling RG, Gilmore R et al. (1993) Intraarterial use of sodium methohexital for provocative testing during brain embolotherapy. AJNR 14: 171-174

Purdy PD (1991) Imaging cerebral blood flow in interventional neuroradiology: Choice of technique and indications. AJNR 12: 424-427

Purdy PD, Batjer HH, Samson D (1991) Management of hemorrhagic complications from preoperative embolization of arteriovenous malformations. J Neurosurg 74: 205-211

Rauch RA, Vinuela F, Dion J et al. (1992) Preembolization functional evaluation in brain arteriovenous malformations: The ability of superselective amytal test to predict neurologic dysfunction before embolization. AJNR 13: 309-314

Sharbrough FW, Messick JM, Sundt TM (1973) Correlation of continuous electroencephalograms with cerebral blood flow during carotid endarterectomy. Stroke 4: 674-683

Spetzler RF, Martin NA (1986) A proposed grading system for arteriovenous malformations. J Neurosurg 65: 476-483

Spetzler RF, Martin NA, Carter LP et al. (1987) Surgical management of large AVMs by staged embolization and operative excision. J Neurosurg 67: 17-28

Spetzler RF, Wilson CB, Weinstein P et al. (1978) Normal perfusion pressure breakthrough theory. Clin Neurosurg 25: 651-672

Steed DL, Webster MW, DeVries EJ et al. (1990) Clinical observations on the effect of carotid artery occlusion on cerebral blood flow mapped by xenon computed tomography and its correlation with carotid artery back pressure. J Vasc Surg 11: 38-44

Taormina MA, Nichols FT (1996) Use of transcranial Doppler sonography to evaluate patients with cerebrovascular disease. In: Meyer FB (ed.) Cerebral blood flow. Neurosurgery Clinics of North America vol 7, pp 589-603

Therapeutics and Technology Assessment Subcommittee of the American Academy of Neurology (1990) Assessment: intraoperative neurophysiology. Neurology 40: 1644-1646

Thomas ML, Walters HL (1980) Hemiplegia as a complication of therapeutic embolization of the internal maxillary artery (abstract). AJNR 1: 283

Valdueza JM, Eckert B, Zanella FE (1994) Detection of MCA embolization during transcranial Doppler monitoring. Neurol Res 16: 137-140

Verhaegen M, Warner DS (1995) Brain protection and brain death. In: Van Aken H (ed.) Neuroanaesthetic practice. BMA Publishing Group, London, pp 267-293

Vinuela F, Debrun G, Fox AJ et al. (1982) Therapeutic embolization of 54 large arteriovenous malformations of the brain with isobutyl-2-cyanoacrylate. Can J Neurol Sci 9: 279

Wada J, Rasmussen T (1960) Intracarotid injection of sodium amytal for the lateralization of speech dominance. Experimental and clinical observations. J Neurosurg 17: 266-281

Werner C, Kochs E (1995) Intraoperative and postoperative monitoring of the CNS for neurosurgery. In: Van Aken H (ed.) Neuroanaesthetic practice. BMA Publishing Group, London, pp 50-181

Westmoreland BF, Klass DW, Sharbrough FW et al. (1975) Alpha coma: electroencephalographic, clinical, pathologic and etiologic correlations. Arch Neurol 32: 713-718

Witt J-P, Yonas H, Jungreis C (1994) Cerebral blood flow response pattern during balloon test occlusion of the internal carotid artery. AJNR 15: 847-857

Yonas H, Linskey M, Johnson DW et al. (1992) Internal carotid balloon test occlusion does require quantitative CBF. AJNR 13: 1147-1148

Yonas HY, Pindzola RR, Johnson DW (1996) Xenon/computed tomography cerebral blood flow and its use in clinical management. In: Meyer FB (ed.) Cerebral Blood Flow. Neurosurgery Clinics of North America vol 7, pp 605-616

Young WL, Pile-Spellman J (1994) Anesthetic considerations for interventional neuroradiology. Anesthesiology 80: 427-456

Zentner J (1989) Noninvasive motor evoked potential monitoring during neurosurgical operations on the spinal cord. Neurosurgery 24: 709-712

Chapter 9
Radiation Therapy and Vascular Malformations

Piers N. Plowman

Introduction: The History and Rationale of Radiation Therapy for Angiomas

The effects of ionising radiation on normal blood vessels have been observed during high dose radiotherapy dose administration in humans and animals. Lindsay et al. (1962) demonstrated that following the administration of high dose radiation to localised segments of dog abdominal aorta, arteriosclerosis occurred that was indistinguishable from that occurring with advancing age, and the progression of the radiation induced lesions also progressed with time. Rubin and Casaret (1968) described the effects of radiation on the aorta of humans: the wall of the aorta was thickened, in some areas up to 4 mm. The intima was thickened and wrinkled. In some regions, fibrin covered the intimal surface, and in other regions there were mural thrombi. However, the majority of the wall thickening was due to an increase in thickness of the adventitia. The main clinical manifestation of radiation damage to large human blood vessels is spontaneous rupture, occurring 1–7 years after doses of 4000–7000 cGy (Fajardo, 1982; Fajardo & Lee, 1975; Trott, 1991), although thrombosis is the other problem that may arise (Drescher et al., 1984). Rubin and Casaret (1968) draw attention to the damage to the fine vasa vasorum (supplying the large vessel walls with oxygen and nutrition) as a probable primary radiation damage target. The vasa vasorum revealed subintimal infiltration by foamy macrophages or subintimal foamy vacuolation and the frequent formation of fibrin thrombi, which later became organised with fibrosis.

Smaller arteries, and more especially arterioles, show degenerative intimal, medial and adventitial changes in the acute and subacute clinical periods after large doses of ionising radiation. Capillaries fare even worse.

The repair of the acute/subacute radiation damage to blood vessels is by secondary intention (fibrosis) and the consequence of this is to leave the affected blood vessel in an advanced degree of arteriosclerosis or obliterated by endarteritis obliterans (Figure 9.1). Small blood vessels, vasa vasorum and capillaries are most predisposed to this.

The tolerance of blood vessels to radiation is a function of both the dose received and the fractionation by which this total dose is administered. (I will not be discussing the different radiobiological efficacy of high energy particulate radiation

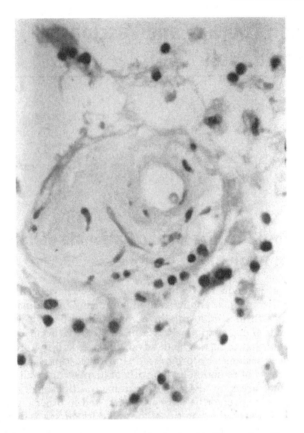

Fig. 9.1. Photomicrograph of radiation-induced endarteritis obliterans of a small artery.

"rad-for-rad" but confining the subsequent discussion to photon radiation; similarly, discussions of ionising radiation delivery dose rates are not considered relevant to this chapter.) This topic is of great importance throughout the subject of normal tissue radiation tolerance as the vasculo-connective tissue's response to higher doses of radiation may be the arbiter of overall tissue tolerance – particularly in "late responding tissues" (e.g. the central nervous system). That blood vessels themselves are late responding tissues to radiation is an observation that may indeed be causal.

When the radiobiologist divides tissues into "early" and "late" responding tissue with regard to radiation tolerance, he does this in the knowledge that different relationships apply with regard to tolerance to dose fractionation. Late responding tissues reach their radiation tolerance level more readily, total dose for total dose, if that radiation dose is delivered in large dose fractions. It follows logically from this that the most damaging way to give radiation to a blood vessels is in a single large dose. We have recently reviewed these radiobiological relationships in more detail (Montefiore & Plowman, 1997).

One other factor that will influence the radiation tolerance of any normal organ is the volume of that tissue irradiated. In general, small volumes tolerate larger doses of radiation than large volumes.

Angiomas and vascular malformations are abnormal vascular structures/tumours in which there is an overgrowth of redundant blood vessels; the constituent blood vessels are not supplying oxygenated blood to any normal tissue. There are various types, which will be discussed below, but only the medullary venous malformation of brain may have a normal functioning blood vessel component. Furthermore, the blood vessels that comprise the abnormality are imperfectly formed, frequently weak-walled and, certainly in the brain, liable to bleed. These abnormalities occur congenitally in the central nervous system or its appendages, although many not maturing to give clinical problems until later in life. Excision or other means of obliteration is curative.

That radiation may obliterate these malformations has been appreciated for some considerable time and it is first interesting to review the efficacy of conventionally fractionated (i.e. relatively low-dose fractions delivered daily) radiotherapy on these growths.

There is evidence that conventionally fractionated doses of radiation will cause remission in angiomas outside the central nervous system/eye. The literature is mainly from paediatric experience and is relevant to discussion of radiotherapeutic obliteration of angiomas of the nervous system which will follow. There are several types of angiomas of childhood. The "strawberry" (capillary) haemangioma presents at birth or soon afterwards (usually in the head and neck region); it may enlarge fast. It has been known for many decades that these angiomas respond dramatically fast following a few small fractions of radiotherapy (e.g. 500 cGy in total) and this is unquestionably the most radiosensitive of all the angioma family (Lister, 1938; Paterson & Todd, 1939; Strandquist, 1939). However, although complete resolution is hastened by radiation, these angiomas spontaneously involute and the radiotherapeutic practice has stopped. Cavernous angiomas are subcutaneous lesions that may arise anywhere in the body (vertebrae, liver, pericardium, orbit, subglottis, etc.) and in the skin they are macular lesions with less definite edges than the strawberry type. Large cavernous haemangiomas may be complicated by the consumption of platelets with sometimes life-threatening thrombocytopenia (Kasabach-Merrit syndrome). Other large haemangiomas may cause high output heart failure due to arteriovenous shunting of blood. Rotman et al. (1980) described the rapid response of such a large hepatic angioma with heart failure to 400 cGy. We have described similar responses to low doses and conventionally fractionated radiation and to steroids of such angiomas (Dutton & Plowman, 1991).

Subglottic angiomas require treatment due to laryngeal obstruction and radiotherapy doses of the order of 400-800 cGy (fractionated) have been successful in causing regression, with prompt relief of stridor and slower resolution of the angioma over weeks to months (Holborow, 1958; Bek et al., 1980). Small initial fraction sizes (40-100 cGy) are used to treat subglottic lesions in the absence of intubation or tracheostomy to reduce the incidence of laryngeal swelling and respiratory distress that occur with the initiation of radiotherapy. The use of radiotherapy, both brachytherapy and external beam therapy in the treatment of ocular angioma is not new (Alberti et al., 1983; Plowman et al., 1988; Greber et al., 1984), nor is the appreciation that these largely cavernous angiomas are more radiosensitive than the retinal capillary angiomas of the von Hippel-Lindau syndrome. The recent impetus to using external beam therapy for ocular angiomas has undoubtedly been fired by more sophisticated technology which allows ocular radiation therapy but with lens and anterior segment sparing (Schipper, 1983; Harnett et al., 1987). In a recently reported series from Essen/Berlin the authors describe good responses to conventionally fractionated radiation to doses as low as 2000 cGy over two weeks (in terms of resolution of subretinal fluid and retinal detachment, although flattening of the angioma – a cause of the visual distortion that these patients suffer – was less reliably affected) (Schilling et al., 1997). In the series reported from London (Barts/Moorfields; Madreperla et al., 1997) similar findings were observed. However, some of the London patients had been treated by brachytherapy (which, in general, delivers higher-dose equivalents of radiation) and when comparing the results of treatment between the conventionally fractionated external beam patients and those treated by brachytherapy they noted that although both groups had a good response of the subretinal fluid and retinal detachment, only the brachytherapy patients obtained flattening of the tumours and improvement of their visual distortion. Zografos et al., (1996) also remain advocates of brachytherapy. The current wisdom at this centre is that circumscribed angiomas are best treated with brachytherapy and diffuse angiomas (as occur in the Sturge–Weber syndrome) are best treated by lens sparing conventionally fractionated external beam therapy. In this latter group we are increasing the prescribed dose to 4000 cGy in order to try to obtain a flattening of the tumour. The observations in the eye work on the different doses needed to stop leakage as opposed to tumour shrinkage are noteworthy (vide infra). We have recently reviewed this subject (Plowman & Hungerford, 1997).

With regard to central nervous system angiomas, the early impressions of efficacy, based on conventionally fractionated radiotherapy, were not favourable (Cushing & Bailey, 1928, Olivercrona & Ladenhim, 1957.) However, Johnson (1979) reviewed 100 cases of cerebral angiomas presenting to Manchester over a 20-year period and found that, following 4000–5000 cGy in 3 weeks. Only 20 patients had a follow-up angiogram but of these, nine patients had been cured and five patients had been improved. There were no complications of therapy. From Brisbane, Poulsen (1987) reported that six cases of inoperable cerebral AVM had been treated with conventionally fractionated radiation and that one patient treated with 7500 cGy in 20 fractions had been cured; the other five patients (modal treatment dose: 5000 cGy in 20 fractions) had not. My own experience with four patients with very large cerebral arteriovenous malformations (AVM) treated to 5000–5500 cGy in 25 fractions is that none have obliterated. I conclude from these data that the efficacy of conventionally fractionated radiation in obliterating cerebral AVM is low, and it is only when the fraction sizes are above 300 cGy and the total doses are in excess of 5000 cGy that there is any real chance of effecting obliteration by standard external beam radiotherapy technology, and even then the chance of obliteration is modest and that this fits with the radiobiological concepts outlined above. However, this is not the case in the eye (after all a central nervous system [CNS] appendage) where, as I have described above, conventionally fractionated radiation has an excellent track record and where it remains one of the standard therapies.

Not often mentioned in the literature is the occasional familial incidence of angiomas. In hereditary haemorrhagic telangiectasia, Osler – Rendu – Weber syndrome) there is an increased risk of bleeding from an AVM and their incidence has been calculated to be 5% (Jesserum et al., 1993; Roman et al., 1978; White et al., 1988; Willinsky et al., 1990; Fulbright et al., 1994). However, in other cases the genetic predisposition does not seem to fit into a recognised syndrome. The following family history is illustrative: a 32-year old lady was referred to this author for radiotherapy to a choroidal haemangioma. She had a past history multiple central nervous system angiographically occult (called cavernous) angiomas, one of which had been surgically excised at craniotomy following a bleed. Her sister had suffered a brain angioma, her son had an incidental discovery of a retinal haemangioma and her father had a buttock cavernous angioma. Although not fitting into recognised syndromes, the not too rare occurrence of multiple arteriovenous malformations is well recognised.

With regard to angiomas and other associated conditions, the Sturge–Weber syndrome is a well-recognised syndrome with facial and central nervous system angiomas and the von Hippel–Lindau syndrome includes ocular and brain haemangioblastomas.

Skeletal haemangiomatosis is another syndrome of relevance to this discussion; the affected patient usually presents with a vertebral lesion(s) with complications. Spinal cord compression has been described (Chrysikopoulos et al., 1996; Plowman, 1997b). There frequently occur multiple vertebral haemangiomas and also visceral ones (e.g. liver). Embolisation and intralesional injections into the vertebral haemangiomas has been reported (Raco et al., 1990; Nicola et al., 1993). The large Mayo Clinic experience of radiotherapy is worthy of note. In this series, young females and the dorsal spine were most at risk of complications including cord damage; radiotherapy in their hands to a conventionally fractionated dose of 30 Gy prevented local progression (Fox et al., 1993).

Radiosurgery for Intracranial Angiomas/Vascular Malformations

With the historical background outlined above, it was not too great a conceptual leap to desire to "focus" radiation therapy doses on targets within the central nervous system. That leap was first made in the 1950s in Sweden by Leksell, albeit not with vascular malformations in mind at the outset. Leksell conceived of image-guided, multiple, cross-firing, small and tightly collimated radiation portals "focusing" a high, single radiotherapy dose on an intracranial target, which in the first endeavours was a functional neurological problem. His original concept was to deliver a single "heavy" dose of radiation to a deep brain structure to destroy that area, without opening the skull; his first clinical work was aimed at destroying intracerebral pathways in functional disorders such as chronic obsessive compulsive states (bearing in mind that this was the era of lobotomy). Leksell conceived the name stereotactic radiosurgery and his idea was to use the narrow focussed beams to replace coagulating electrodes which were then in use in the treatment of pain, Parkinson's disease and other movement disorders (Leksell, 1951). He initiated the high single dose radiotherapy/radiosurgery that is currently practised for CNS angioma therapy (fractionated radiosurgery is reserved for non-angioma work). His early work was hampered by the equipment as only a 200 kV therapy unit was available to him. Nevertheless, the concept was born in those early 1950s and the principle of "focusing" single high doses of radiotherapy within the nervous system for therapeutic effect has now survived four decades of use and remains one of the principal methods of curing brain angiomas currently. The concept was next furthered in Stockholm in 1968 with the introduction of the "Gamma Knife" (Elekta Instruments, Inc, Tucker, GA). Technically, this unit comprises a heavily shielded central body currently containing 201 sources of ^{60}Co. The sources are radially distributed over a segment of the spherical core/head helmet and the beams are individually collimated towards a common point (the stereotactic target) in the centre of the helmet. Standard collimator sizes of 4, 8, 14 and 18 mm are available and their use, singly or in combination, allows lesions of different size and shape to be targeted. A stereotactic three-dimensional dose planning system is used to obtain optimal dosimetry, ensuring the isodose distribution best encompasses the target volume. Single channels can be blocked if a particular normal structure close to the target must be protected. The so-called gamma knife thus maintains the original idea of concentrating a very high radiation dose on the target volume with a very sharp and rapid fall-off at the perimeter.

Other systems have subsequently been developed which achieve comparable dosimetry. Heavy charged particle therapy has the capability of delivering equivalent concentrated doses of therapeutic radiation. Beams of monoenergetic heavy charged particles, such as helium ions, create a depth dose profile of highly concentrated ionising radiation deposition at the end of their path length (the Bragg peak phenomenon). This development was pioneered at the Donner Radiation Laboratory, University of California-Berkeley (Lawrence, 1985). Helium ions have a sharp lateral edge due to a small angle of lateral scatter and this sharp lateral and distal fall-off of dose and the enhanced dose in the Bragg peak region lead to a radiosurgery capability that can challenge other methods (Steinberg et al., 1990). The radiobiological efficacy of helium ions is greater than photons (and a relative biological efficacy [RBE] factor of 1.3 is employed when comparing doses).

The use of standard linear accelerator facilities, utilising their isocentric mounting and rotation technology to create the dose concentration required for radiosurgery by an adaptation of arcing technology, has evolved over the last decade to be a major competing method of radiosurgery (Heifetz et al., 1984). Hartmann et al., (1985) claimed accuracy to within 1 mm and subsequent workers proved that this "x-knife" technology could rival that of the other stereotactic radiosurgical methods (Saunders et al., 1988; Thomson et al., 1990). In these linac methods of radiosurgery, the treatment machine arcs around the target point with the treatment beam only ever pointing at that stereotactically mapped point. At the end of several arcs, the dose accumulated by the target is huge but, at the perimeter of the target, the dose fall-off is comparably fast to other stereotactic radiosurgical methods. In the method described from St. Bartholomew's Hospital (Thomson et al., 1990), a new type of relocatable stereotactic frame was introduced that has led to a versatility in stereotactic radiotherapy that was previously not achievable, namely the capability of routine fractionation.

There are, therefore, three main methods of radiosurgery now available in current clinical practice. A recent critique and comparison of the three techniques is educational, (Phillips et al., 1994). A synopsis of their comparison was that for small lesions (less than 5 cm^3) all the three methods of radiosurgery are comparable dosimetrically. Particle beam and a linear accelerator systems are superior to the gamma knife for intermediate (5–25) cm^3 lesions. The dose distribution of charged particle beam radiosurgery makes this the most useful in treating larger lesions over 25 cm^3. The main disadvantage of the gamma knife at larger target volumes is the larger dose heterogeneity within the treatment volume and the fact that these large-dose gradients created by the multiple isocentre technique that the gamma knife necessarily utilises to treat larger volumes, are closely correlated with the complication rates following treatment (Nedzi et al., 1991). In their conclusion, Phillips et al. state: "As a tool to facilitate advances in areas of dosimetry optimisation, such as dynamic conformal therapy (the moulding of treatment isodoses to the target volume), the linac system is the most promising". I would agree with this and the development of micro-multileaf collimator technology in recent years is bringing this prediction true (Schlegel et al., 1997).

Orthogonal plane high resolution angiography, within the stereotactic frame (with evaluation of early arterial and late venous phases) is the backbone of AVM radiosurgery planning, no matter what technology is used for treatment. MR imaging is limited in its differentiation of arterial nidus from venous elements and MR compatible stereotactic frames have only now materialised. Nevertheless, MR/CT can provide useful additional information - for example the third dimension given by MR - and the ability to fuse images in modern planning software makes it easier to assimilate data from different technologies into the final planning decisions.

Steiner et al. (1994) reported the follow-up of 880 patients with high flow AVM using the gamma knife and an intended marginal dose of 2500 cGy; 89% of the patients had been referred because of haemorrhage. Four hundred and sixty-one had a 2-year follow-up angiogram. Three hundred and sixty-nine AVM (80%) were totally obliterated by this 2-year time-point. Obliteration of the AVM within 1 year of therapy occurred in 230 of 360 studied patients. The authors continued to see obliterations after 2 years. Subsequent work seems to show that higher doses lead to faster obliteration rates, but it is certainly true that sclerosis of AVM can continue after 2 years in a minority of patients and so this warns against too early alternative therapy.

The definition of obliteration needs a moment thought. Linquist and Steiner (1988) define this as: angiographic appearance with normal circulation time, complete absence of pathological vessels in the former nidus and the disappearance or normalisation of draining veins from the area. Steinberg et al. (1990) defined obliteration as the absence of any angiographically visible arteriovenous shunt. The definition must be strict if results are to be comparable.

Steiner et al. (1994) also noted that the efficacy of treatment was related to the volume of the AVM and to the dose received to the periphery of the nidus. When a dose of 2500 cGy was delivered to the periphery of an AVM of up to 1 cm^3, the incidence of obliteration was 88%, when up to 3 cm^3 the obliteration rate was 78%, and in AVM up to 4–8 cm^3 the obliteration rate was 50%. When the peripheral dose was a lower one of 1600–2400 cGy the obliteration rate of AVM with a nidus diameter of 1–3 cm^3 was 70%, which initially implied to these authors a slightly lower obliteration rate. However, interestingly, when the larger AVM (4–8 cm^3) that had been treated by 1600–2400 cGy were scrutinised, they found that 14 of 128 (78%) had been obliterated, suggesting to this author that there not much difference in cure rate between these two dosages with regard to ultimate chance of obliteration.

Steiner et al. (1994) also analysed the results of treating AVM in children. One hundred and six children had undergone a 2-year angiogram after radiosurgery and 88 had completely obliterated (83%) with no improvement in only 3%. The technique is undoubted indicated in children as in adults.

Another aspect of their study was to examine the efficacy and safety of retreating AVM that had not completely obliterated after two to three years from radiosurgery. In 97 such patients they had retreated and then found that 33 of 40 (87.6%) had subsequently totally sclerosed. It is implied that such retreatment carries low morbidity risks and they quote a 5% permanent complication rate in their manuscript, which compares to their 3% permanent complication rate for first time treatment; this is an important aspect to further research. In the Sheffield experience, using the gamma knife, as did Steiner et al., I am informed that the retreatment risks are not significantly higher than after first time therapy (D. Forster, personal communication). I think it is probably the case that the retreating clinicians have very carefully retreated a smaller/shrunken nidus to a conservative retreatment dose and got away without problems. Whilst the Charlottesville/Karolinska (Steiner et al., 1994) and Sheffield data are, therefore, at first very encouraging for the re-use of radiosurgery to an incompletely sclerosed AVM nidus; nevertheless; all practitioners should caution great care in this situation.

A last subgroup analysis carried out by Steiner et al. was to examine the efficacy of combined embolisation and radiosurgery. Two hundred and fourteen patients had embolisation followed by radiosurgery. Two-year follow-up angiography had been performed in only 32 cases. Total obliteration had occurred in 17 (53%) patients. If only the 23 optimally treated (not defined) cases were considered, the total obliteration rate was 17/23 (74%). Lastly in the Steiner et al. (1994) analysis, we are informed that 5–8 year angiogram had been performed in 30 patients who had been deemed cured at the 2-year angiogram time-point, and that none showed recanalisation. It is clear that radiosurgery cure of an AVM at the 2-year angiogram time-point is a permanent one.

It would be re-assuring to know that this fact remains true for the combined embolisation/radiosurgery series, but I suspect that the data are not mature enough for us to know that with certainty yet; the potential problems with combined embolisation/radiosurgery are further discussed below.

The Pittsburgh gamma knife group reported the early follow-up of 227 AVM patients treated with a mean marginal dose of 21.2 Gy (range 12–27 Gy) in a single radiosurgery session, but with the intention to deliver a dose of 20 Gy at least to the margin of the nidus where it was deemed safe to do so. Seventy-five patients had been followed for more than two years and of those who had repeated angiography at this point, the obliteration rates were: 8/8 (100%) of AVM less than 1 cm^3, 22/26 (85%) of nidus diameter 1–4 cm^3, and 7/12 (58%) of nidus diameter more than 4 cm^3. From what can only be described as an early analysis, these data from Pittsburgh seem to concur with the larger Charlottesville data. Ten patients from their whole series had suffered a repeat haemorrhage in the interval to obliteration.

Linear-accelerator-based radiosurgery results have been presented by several groups and I will first present the St. Bartholomew's group data here. Between March 1989 and December 1993, 101 patients were referred to the radiosurgical service at St. Bartholomew's Hospital. All patients were treated with a uniform dose of 1750 cGy, prescribed to the 90% isodose which circumscribed the nidus (the marginal dose). Fifty-two patients had follow-up angiography at the time of analysis (Sebag-Montefiore et al., 1995). The complete obliteration rates were 75–77% for AVM up to 10 cm^3 (25 mm) and 45–75% for AVM over 10 cm^3, when studied 18–30 months after radiosurgery. These figures have been maintained with more patients and longer follow-up. The problem of haemorrhage in the interval to obliteration was studied. Four patients developed haemorrhage following treatment and prior to obliteration. Two patients rebled early at 4 and 7 months; they both fully recovered and went on to completely obliterate by 22 and 32 months respectively. Of the two patients who rebled later (at 18 and 20 months) the first required emergency evacuation of haematoma, from which there was fully recovery, but the other patient died of intraventricular haemorrhage. The two year risk of rebleeding (a sensible time-point statistic in that the majority of AVM have obliterated by then) was 5.1% in this London series. These data are similar to those from Vicenza (Colombo et al., 1993) where the obliteration rate at 2 years was a similar 80% using a comparable linear accelerator technique.

The Barts group also studied the influence of treatment on the epilepsy associated with AVM (Falkson et al., 1997). They were not the first group to look at this aspect: 24% of patients presenting to Barts with AVM gave a history of epilepsy (which is similar to the presenting incidences reported by others: Duruty et al., 1994 who reported 31%, Steiner et al., 1992 who reported 24% and Sutcliffe et al., 1992 who reported their patients' incidence to be 40%. In the first 101 patients presenting to Barts with symptomatic AVM, there 24 patients with a history of prior epilepsy.

Eight were non-evaluable. Of 16 evaluable patients, 15/16 (94%) had improvement of their fit control, 10/16 (63%) becoming fit-free. This improvement appeared to correlate with response to treatment on angiography and in 11/15 patients this occurred with no change or a reduction in anti-convulsant medication. No patient suffered a deterioration in the epilepsy. These data supported the observations of others that radiosurgical treatment of AVM improves the associated epilepsy; thus Steiner et al. (1992) reported that 70% of patients gained improvement of their fit control following treatment and Sutcliffe et al. (1992) 60% improvement, 38% with no further fits. In the discussion of these observations, Falkson et al. theorise that the improvement is due an alteration in the "scar" caused by the lesion within the brain or a change in the regional blood flow caused by the successful treatment of the AVM. In comments that followed that publication, Kurita (1997) drew attention to the fact that a similar reduction in epileptic severity had been noted in patients with tumour related epilepsy.(Rogers et al., 1993; Rossi et al., 1985) and also described his own observations in Tokyo of an improvement in the fit control earlier than the response of AVM angiographically – he described improvement as early as the first few months after therapy which would not have been expected on regional blood flow reasoning based on angiography (Kurita et al., 1997; Kurita, 1997). Plowman (1997) replied that the Barts group had observed changes in blood flow on SPET scans earlier than they could be detected on angiograms (indeed Kashyap et al., [1996] had suggested that SPECT scanning could be used early after radiosurgery to predict success on this basis) and so the theory that amelioration of the shunt through the AVM, resulting in improvement of regional blood flow to normal brain could still be the mechanism of the improvement in the epilepsy. Plowman pointed out that the new imaging technique of phase contrast MRA may be a future method of sorting this interesting mechanistic problem out – further work is obviously needed. A major reason for wanting to sort out this problem is that it impacts on functional radiosurgery for intractable seizures and the rationale for this.

Another aspect of the St. Bartholomew's experience which is worthy of debate is the use of radiosurgery in larger AVM. With the linear accelerator technology, it is possible to more homogenously radiosurgically treat larger AVM, say up to 35–40 mm diameter, and the data are now accumulating on the cure rates if this practice: Sebag-Montefiore et al. (1995) reported the obliteration of 7/14 (50%) of AVM larger than 25 mm diameter and Engenhardt et al. (1994) reporting the Heidelberg linear accelerator experience agree with this figure of 50% for the larger AVM also, whereas Colombo et al. (1993) found only a 33% obliteration rate for AVM above 25 mm diameter (10 cm^3). It seems clear that the larger the AVM diameter/volume the more difficult it is to obliterate, particularly bearing in mind that normal tissue tolerance considerations make it essential to dose reduce as the nidus diameter/volume increases to a large size. Proton beam data (vide infra) are also in accord with these observations. Nevertheless, the point remains that for these large AVM which are problematic to surgeons and embolisers too, radiosurgery may cure a substantial fraction of the population (Figure 9.2). The experience with embolisation has been less in our hospital than that reported by Steiner, although it will be noted that that data is difficult to interpret because of the relatively small number of follow-up data at the time of analysis, the undefined term "optimally treated", and the relatively short space of manuscript devoted to it. In our experience, which includes 17 patients in the first 100 who had received embolisation prior to radiosurgery, it was clear that embolisation often took the central part of the nidus away. This satisfactorily reduced the vascularity of the AVM but it

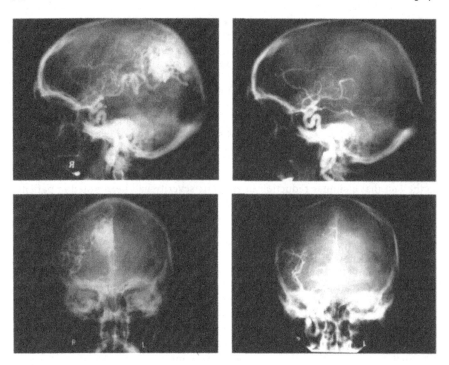

Fig. 9.2. Angiograms before (left panels) and after (right panels) radiosurgery for a large AVM that was cured by the procedure.

could well leave the overall nidus diameter (radiosurgical target volume) unchanged. A far more satisfactory approach is one where the interventional radiologist and the radiosurgery clinicians can form a strategy (perhaps easiest where there is an irregular shaped, say comet shape, AVM whose blood supply favours embolisation to eliminate the comet tail and then radiosurgery has a more discrete nidus to target) to reduce the morbidities of both procedures and gain the benefits of each. What strikes this author as folly is to embolise the epicentre (with the attendant risks of that procedure) and then give radiosurgery (with its attendant risks) to an undiminished overall nidus diameter, because the embolisation has not reduced the overall diameter of the nidus. This is just adding procedural risks.

Similar results have been reported using heavy charged particle beams to treat AVM. Using the Bragg peak of helium ions, the Berkeley Laboratory group reported treating 86 AVM patients with doses of 8.8–34.6 Gy delivered to volumes of tissue of 0.3–70 cm^3. Two years after treatment, the complete obliteration rate was 94% for lesions smaller than 4 cm^3, 75% for lesions of 4–25 cm^3 and 39% for lesions larger than 25 cm^3. Major neurological complications occurred in 10 patients of whom 8 had permanent deficits. All these complications occurred in the initial stage of the protocol before the dose was reduced to 19.2 Gy; the authors concluded that their early doses of up to 34.6 Gy risked morbidity to normal tissues (Steinberg et al. 1990). Levy from the Berkeley group, reported that children responded better than the elderly in their experience – 17/17 had obliterated following radiosurgery (Levy, 1992) and this fits with our early data also (Sebag-Montefiore et al., 1994).

The subject of complications following a radiosurgery for AVM is a very important one. Steiner et al. (1994) found CT changes, indicative of radiation oedema or damage, in the surrounding normal nervous tissue (and the distinction between these two is critical in that the former is usually reversible) in 11% of patients and later this figure rose to 37% when MRI became the follow-up imaging modality. The mean latency of onset between treatment and the onset of radiation induced changes in the surrounding normal nervous system was 9.9 months (range 4-42 months) and this resolved between 1-29 months (mean 9.5 months). However, only 6% of patients were symptomatic from these changes and only 3% suffered permanent complications (Steiner et al., 1994). In Lunsford's series (gamma knife with a mean marginal dose of 21.2 Gy), 10/227 (4.4%) developed new neurological deficits, two of which appeared permanent giving a rate of just under 1%. However, as in Steiner's series, radiological (CT/MR) evidence of oedema in the surrounding brain was found in 24%, high signal changes on T2 weighted images, low density on CT) (Lunsford et al., 1991). Sutcliffe et al. (1992) reported 6/167 (3.5%) patients developing permanent complications following gamma knife radiosurgery in Sheffield (25-50 Gy). Two of these six patients had pontine AVM and four had AVM with nidus diameters of greater than 3 cm; unfortunately the reader is not informed as to the total number of larger AVM treated in that series. In the proton series (Steinberg et al. 1990), 10/20 (50%) of patients receiving doses above 1800 cGy to volumes greater than 13 cm^3, developed major or minor complications. These were the first data to demonstrate clearly a volume effect, as most gamma knife series had concentrated on small nidus cases. As already stated above, this proton group also demonstrated that the complication rate was a function of the size of the single radiosurgery dose delivered.

In our own analysis of 101 patients receiving radiosurgery at St. Bartholomew's Hospital, we found an actuarial risk of 1.8% for permanent neurological deficits in patients with nidus diameter of less than 25 mm (10 cm^3), as compared to 16% incidence in 36 patients with nidus diameter of greater than 25 mm. These are the hardest data available demonstrating a volume effect in photon radiosurgery, as all the patients were treated with one (relatively conservative) dose prescription and by a photon technique with a relatively small internal dose gradient within the target volume (in contrast to gamma knife series). Thus, the Barts data for large AVM suggest a 40% cure rate that has to be set beside an anticipated complication rate of 16% (Sebag-Montefiore et al., 1995); these data have prompted us to move to a research study of a biological response modifier to ameliorate the risk of radiation damage in the treatment of larger AVM; the results are pending.

In summary, the complication rate is related to volume, dose and technique (and differences in technique related to both differences in the relative biological effectiveness [RBE] of the ionising radiation used and the internal dose gradient generated within the treatment volume and the fall-off of the dose at the margin). Most of the early gamma knife data applied to small AVM (less than 5 cm^3), but with linear accelerator and proton radiosurgery, it is now possible to more safely treat larger AVM without the huge internal dose gradients that accompany the gamma knife technology. However, there is still a larger risk factor involved and the clinical questions that arise relate to whether prior surgery or embolisation can reduce the volume to be treated without adding to overall treatment risks and whether a biological response modifier for normal nervous tissue could improve the benefit to risk ratio.

Angiographically Occult Vascular Malformations

Angiographically occult vascular malformations (AOVM) include a variety of pathological entities associated with two imaging hallmarks: well-defined areas of abnormal signal with a surrounding haemosiderin deposit, well seen on MR images but no angiographically demonstrable lesion. Pathological examination of AOVM reveal patent or thrombosed arteriovenous malformation or cavernous angioma: occasionally, they may be capillary telangiectasis or rarely venous (as in medullary venous) malformations. The pathological heterogeneity and the diverse clinical manifestations have been emphasised by many authors (Wakai et al., 1985; Simard et al., 1986; Tagle et al., 1986; Ebeling et al., 1988; Lobato et al., 1988; Ogilvy et al., 1988; Yasargi et al., 1988; Kashiwaga et al., 1990; Kondziolka et al., 1990, 1995a). Whilst some authors consider cavernous angiomas to account for the vast majority of AOVM, other authors find that cryptic AVM comprise a larger proportion (Wakai et al., 1985). Since the advent of high quality MRI, a higher proportion of these vascular malformations are being correctly labelled as cavernous malformations. However, the tendency by some authors to use the term cavernous angioma for all AOVM is not always correct, as Kondziolka et al. (1995a) point out, there is a differential diagnosis which includes the other possible causes outlined above.

Histologically, the true cavernous angioma is characterised by dilated thin-walled vascular channels lined by a simple endothelium and thin fibrous adventitia; no brain substance nor normal blood vessels (i.e. blood carrying oxygenated blood to or from normal brain) is contained within the angioma. However, interestingly, there is an occasional associated medullary venous malformation associated with the cavernous angioma (Wilms et al., 1994; Scamoni et al., 1997), and as medullary venous angioma may have a normal vasculature (a physiological venous drainage component) this is important to recognise as surgical or radiosurgical treatment of the medullary venous component risks complications.Whilst many AOVM remain silent clinically and are nowadays diagnosed more often incidentally on MRI taken for other reasons, nevertheless, some are prone to multiple bleeds and worsening morbidity with each bleed.

Radiosurgery results of AOVM treatment have been reported by several large institutions; Kondziolka et al. (1990) reported 24 patients treated by gamma knife radiosurgery for haemorrhaging AOVM. Nineteen patients either improved or remained stable with no further haemorrhage, whilst one patient had further haemorrhage. Five patients suffered delayed complications, in two of whom these were serious although in one of these two a deteriorating neurological baseline prior to treatment was maintained following the treatment and so the cause of the ongoing problem was not clear.

Levy et al. (1992) reported 31 patients treated by proton radiosurgery for AOVM because of haemorrhage or mass effect; only six had rebled after treatment. Two patients with brainstem lesions suffered radiation induced neurological damage. Of the others, two patients suffered temporary sequelae that fully resolved with steroid therapy.

Kondziolka et al. (1995b) updated their 1990 analysis of response data to radiosurgery for AOVM. Of 47 patients who received radiosurgery for bleeding AOVM the rebleeding risk was dramatically reduced. With regard to complications, there was an interesting early transient morbidity which settled on steroid therapy, in up to 20–25% of the patients, but only two patients had new permanent neurological damage. The doses that these Pittsburgh workers recommend are marginal doses of 10–20 Gy with maximum doses in the range 20–40 Gy.

Kida et al. (1996) reported 51 cases of symptomatic AOVM. Of 37 cases presenting with haemorrhage, 32 showed no further haemorrhage after radiosurgery. Of 11 patients presenting with intractable seizures, seven demonstrated good seizure control and the other four showed no change in fit frequency. Follow-up imaging showed no obvious change on MRI in 29 patients, shrinkage in 18 patients and enlargement in three patients. Nine patients demonstrated neurological symptoms within 12 months of treatment but after steroid therapy only two patients suffered long-term neurological morbidity.

In their discussion, Kida et al. conclude, as indeed the synthesis of the foregoing leads us, that "persistent bleeders" and "refractory fitters" with AOVM should be considered for radiosurgery. The authors recommend a marginal dose of 1700 cGy to supratentorial lesions and 1500 cGy to brainstem lesions.

The predominance of brainstem and difficult, inoperable, deep sites for AOVM referred for radiosurgery and the possibility of co-existing medullary venous angioma should be considered prior to radiosurgery for AOVM and this author agrees with the conservative dose prescriptions just suggested. With such therapy, there are now convincing data that radiosurgery reduces the rehaemorrhage risk; it is presumed that the radiation induced damage to the blood vessel walls is similar to that received by AVMs.

Arteriovenous Dural Fistulae

These lesions are nowadays regarded as acquired lesions, with the neurovascular network often occurring subsequent to injury or thrombosis. Many are incidental findings and may not need therapy. Whilst these lesions may be confined to the dura and fed by dural blood vessels, they may involve both the dura and the brain draining blood supply from dural and pial vessels. Typically, there is a nidus of small fistulae within the dural wall of a venous sinus – fed arterially by a dural artery. Sometimes there is a direct arterial feeder into a dural sinus – the most striking example being the carotid–cavernous fistula. The dural sinus is the sole drainage in most cases but cortical veins may contribute in tentorial fistulae. It is this normal vasculature that pleads for great care in the therapy of symptomatic cases.

As discussed elsewhere in this text, transarterial superselective embolisation of the feeding artery may effect cure or thereabout; but the venous route, placing coils or other embolic material in the draining sinus may also be effective if safe to do so – occlusion of a dural sinus with retrograde flow of blood in the cortical veins risking venous infarction or haemorrhage being a risk.

Radiosurgical experience in the treatment of arteriovenous fistulae is limited at present, but the data that have been published are of interest and some is persuasive. Steiner et al. (1994) had 2-year angiographic follow-up on 11 small fistulae (nidus diameter up to 2.5 cm). Three had totally obliterated and one partially; one patient rebled and was retreated and subsequently obliterated. None of eight larger fistulae obliterated in this series, which implies to this author that surgery or embolisation should precede radiosurgery where possible.

The carotid–carvernous fistula is a special case with the proptosis, ophthalmoplegia and chemosis, with or without facial pain, being memorable physical signs. The radiosurgical experience here is slightly greater and firmer. Steiner et al. (1994) reported treating eight patients, four of whom had adequate follow-up to analyse. All four had obliterated. Moriki et al., 1993 reported the obliteration of two of two carotid–cavernous fistulae by radiosurgery.

Barcia-Solero et al. (1994) reported 25 patients with carotid-cavernous fistulae treated by gamma knife radiosurgery (to 30-40 Gy). Of 22 spontaneous fistulae, 20/22 (91%) closed completely without recurrence by 1.3-14 years (mean time to closure ~7.5 months), with clinical improvement being noted at a mean of 2.4 months (a surprising early time). In this Spanish series, there were three traumatic, high-flow fistulae and only one of these obliterated following radiosurgery (and this one closed by 6 months). There were no complications to treatment in this series.

Thus the synthesis of what data there are suggest that, most persuasively for the lower flow rate carotid-cavernous fistulae, that radiosurgery is an attractive first-line definitive therapy with a low complication rate.

Glomus Jugulare Tumours

There is a good body of literature on the efficacy of conventionally fractionated radiation on glomus jugulare tumours. Local control rates of 85-100% have been reported (Cole and Beiler, 1994; Larner et al., 1992; Powell et al., 1992; Schild et al., 1992; Skolyszewski et al., 1991; Springate et al., 1991) with a complication rate of less than 10%. It therefore seemed appropriate to use radiosurgery in this discrete and non-malignant tumour.

The Mayo Clinic have recently reported on nine glomus jugulare tumours treated by gamma knife technology (1800 cGy to two small tumours up to 7 cc, 1500 cGy to four intermediate tumours and 1200 cGy to three tumours of greater than 11.5 cc volume). With a median time to analysis of 20 months (range 7-65) there was improvement in symptoms in 7/9, stability in size in 8/9 on MR and reduction in size in one patient's tumour; there were no compications (Foot et al., 1997). These Mayo Clinic authors, and I agree with them, conclude that this is the optimal means of radiotherapy in most instances.

Venous Angiomas (syn. Medullary Venous Angioma)

As agonised above with regard to the normal tissue components of arteriovenous dural fistulae, the venous component of a venous angioma contains a normal physiological venous component. Thus although Steiner et al. (1994) reported on radiosurgery to the "caput medusae" in 13 patients, their results were poor (1/12 analysable patients cured) and 4/13 patients developed complications (a rate that surgeons encounter with excision of these growths – probably due to the physiological/normal vessel component). Radiosurgery is not currently recommended for these angiomas.

Arterial Aneurysms

Although not standard practice, or ever likely to be, and this author has no experience at all, Steiner et al. (1994) report treating nine aneurysms by radiosurgery and obliterating 3/5 assessable cases. In the gamma knife data bank of cases treated and, as of June 1997, I was interested to see that 90 cases of aneurysm had received this treatment and it would be important to pool and examine the results.

References

Alberti W, Greber H, John V, Wessing A, Scherer E (1983) Radiotherapy of the hemangioma of the choroid. Strahlentherapie 159: 160-167

Barcia-Salorio JL, Soler F, Barcia JA, Hernandez G (1994) Radiosurgery of carotid-cavernous fistulae. Acta Neurochir Suppl. 62: 10-12

Bek V, Abrahamova J, Koutecky J, Kolihova E, Fajstar J (1980) Perinatal subglottic and hepatic hemangiomas as potential emergencies: effect of radiotherapy, Neoplasma 27: 337-344

Chrsikopoulos H, Roussakis A, Tsakkraklides V, Vassilouthis J (1996) Case report: sclerotic skeletal haemangiomatosis presenting with spinal cord compression - CT and MRI findings. Br J Radiol 69: 965-967

Cole JM, Beiler D (1994) Long-term results of treatment for glomus jugulare and glomus vagale tumor with radiotherapy. Laryngoscope 104(12): 1461-5

Colombo F, Pozza F, Chierego G, Casenti L (1993) Linear accelerator radiosurgery of cerebral arteriovenous malformations: current status. Acta Neurochir (Wien) 122: 136

Cushing H, Bailey P (1928) Tumors arising from the blood vessels of the brain. Angiomatous malformations and hemangioblastoma. Charles C Thomas, Springfield, p 219

Drescher W, Basche S, Schumann E (1989) Arterielle Spaetkomplikationen nah strahlentherapie. Strahlentherapie 160: 505-507

Duruty R, Pellisou-Guyorat I, Mottolese C (1994) Prognostic value of Spetzler's grading system in a series of cerebral AVM treated by combined management. Acta Neurchir (Wien) 131: 169-175

Dutton SC, Plowman PN (1991) Paediatric haemangiomas: the role of radiotherapy. Br J Radiol 64: 261-269

Ebeling JD, Tranmer BI, Davis KA, Kindt GW, DeMasters BK (1988) Thrombosed arteriovenous malformations: a type of occult vascular malformation. Neurosurgery 23: 605-610

Fajardo LF (1982) Pathology of radiation injury. Masson, New York

Fajardo LF, Lee HA (1975) Rupture of major vessels after radiation. Cancer 36: 904-913

Falkson CB, Chakraborti KB, Doughty D, Plowman PN (1997) Stereotactic multiple arc radiotherapy - influence of treatment of arteiovenous malformations on associated epilepsy. Br J Neurosurg 11: 12-15

Foot RL, Coffey RJ, Gorman DA, Earle JD, Schomberg PJ, Kline RW, Schild SE (1997) Stereotactic radiosurgery for glomus jugulare tumors: a preliminary report. Int J Radiat Biol Phys 38(3): 491-5

Fox MW, Onofrio BM (1993) The natural history and management of symptomatic and asymptomatic vertebral haemangiomas. J Neurosurg 78: 36-45

Fulbright RK, Merriam MA, Fayad PB, Sze GK, Egglin TK, White RI (1994) Hereditary haemorrhagic telangiectasia: correlation of MR imaging and clinical findings in 130 patients. Radiology 193: Suppl. 211 Abstract

Greber H, Wessing A, Alberti W, Scherer E (1984) Successful treatment of choroidal hemangioma with secondary changes caused by the Sturge - Weber syndrome. Klin Monatsbl Augenheilkd 185: 276-278

Harnett A, Hungerford J, Lambert G et al. (1987) Improved external beam therapy for the treatment of retinoblastoma. Br J Radiol 60: 753-760

Heifetz MD, Wexler M, Thompson R (1984) Single beam radiotherapy knife. J Neurosurg 60: 814-818

Hartmann GH, Schlegel W, Sturm V, Kober B, Pastyr O, Lorenz Wj (1985) Cerebral radiation surgery using moving field irradiation at a linear accelerator facility. Int J Radiat Oncol 11: 1185-1192

Holborow CA (1958) Subglottic hemangiomas: two infants with laryngeal stridor. Arch Dis Child 33: 210-211

Jesserum GAJ, Kamphius DJ, van der Zande FHR, Nossent JC (1993) Cerebral arteriovenous malformations in the Netherlands Antilles: high prevalence of hereditary haemorrhegic telangiectasia related single and multiple cerebral arteriovenous malformations. Clin Neurol Neurosurg 95: 193-198

Johnson RT (1974) Radiotherapy of cerebral angiomas with a note on on some problems in diagnosis. In: Pia HW, Gleave JRW, Grote E, Zierski J (eds) Cerebral angiomas, advances in diagnosis and therapy. Springer-Verlag, Berlin, pp 256-266

Kashiwaga S, Van Loveren HR, Tew JM, Wiot JG, Weil SM, Lukin RA (1990) Diagnosis and treatment of vascular branstem malformations. J Neurosurg 72: 27-34

Kashyap R, Carroll MJ, Huneidi AHS, Nimmon C, Plowman PN, Britton KE (1996) Quantitative cerebral blood flow analysis in predicting radiosurgical outcome of cerebral AVM. Nucl Med Comm 17: 299 abstract

Kida Y, Koboyashi T, Tanaka T (1996) Radiosurgery of symptomatic angiographically occult vascular malformations with gamma knife. In: Kondziolka D (ed.) Radiosurgery 1995 Vol 1 Karger, Basel pp 207-217

Kondziolka D, Lunsford D, Coffey RJ, Bissonette DJ, Flickinger JC (1990) Sterotactic radiosurgery of angiographically occult vascular malformations: indications and preliminary experience. Neurosurgery 27: 892-900

Kondziolka D, Lunsford D, Kestle JRW (1995a) The natural history of cerebral cavernous malformations. J Neurosurg 83: 820-824

Kondziolka D, Lunsford LD, Flickinger JC, Kestle JRW (1995b) Reduction of hemorrhage risk after stereotactic radiosurgery for carvenous malformations. J Neurosurg 83: 825-831

Kurita H, Suzuki I, Kawamoto S, Sasaki T, Kirino T, Tago M (1997) Seizure outcome in patients with radisurgically treated arteriovenous malformations. Abstract of the 12th Meeting of the World Society for stereotactic and functional radiosurgery, Lyon, France, 1997

Kurita H (1997) Stereotactic radiotherapy for arteriovenous malformations. Br J Neurosurg 11: 591-592

Larner JM, Hahn SS, Spaulding CA, Constable WC (1992) Glomus jugulare tumors. Long-term control by radiation therapy. Cancer 69(7): 1813-7

Lawrence JH (1985) Heavy particle radiation of intracranial lesions. In: Wilkens Rh, Rengachary SS (eds) Neurosurgery. McGraw Hill, New York, pp 1113-1132

Leksell L (1951) The stereotaxic method and radiosurgery of the brain Acta Chir Scand 102: 316

Levy RP (1992) Communication in Editor's comments on radiosurgery in vascular malformations: Steiner L (ed) Radiosurgery. Baseline and Trends. Raven Press, New York, pp 229-223

Lindquist C, Steiner L (1988) Stereotactic radiosurgical treatment of malformations of the brain. In: Lunsford LD (ed.) Modern stereotactic neurosurgery. Martinus Nijhoff, Boston, pp 491-505

Lindsay S, Kohn HI, Dakin RL, Jew J (1962). Aortic arteriosclerosis in he dog after localised aortic x-irradiation. Circ Res 10: 51-67

Lister WA (1938) The natural history of strawberry naevi. Lancet 1: 1429-1434

Lobato RD, Perez C, Rivos JJ, Cordobes F (1988) Clinical, radiological and pathological spectrum of angiographically occult vascular malformations: analysis of 21 cases and review of the literature. J Neurosurg 68: 518-531

Lunsford LD, Kondziolka D, Flickinger JC et al. (1991) Stereotactic radiosurgery for arteriovenous malformations of the brain. J Neurosurg 75: 512-524

Madreperla S, Hungerford JL, Plowman PN (1997) Choroidal hemangiomas: treatment by photocoagulation or radiotherapy. Ophthalmology 104: 1773-1779

Montefiore D, Plowman PN. Clinical applications of radiiotherapy. In: Pinkerton R, Plowman PN (eds) Paediatric oncology Chapman Hall, London, pp 147-158

Moriki A, Mori T, Makino A, et al. (1993) The successful treatment of two carotid-cavernous fistula cases using the gamma knife. Acta Neurochir (Wien) 122: 140 Abstr. 20

Nedzi LA, Kooy H, Alexander E (1991) Variables associated with the development of complications from radiosurgery of intracranial tumours. Int J Radiat Oncol 21: 591-599

Nicola N, Lins E (1993) Vertebral hemangioma. Late results of retrograde embolisation - stabilisation with methyl methacrylate in two cases. Surg Neurol 40: 491-494

Ogilvy CS, Heros RC, Ojemann RG, New PF (1988) Angiographically occult arteriovenous malformations. J Neurosurg 69: 350-355

Olivercrona H, Ladenhim J (1957) Congenital arteriovenous aneurysms of the carotid and vertebral systems. Springer Verlag, Berlin.

Peterson R, Todd MC (1939) The radium treatment of angioma in children. Am J Roentgenol 42: 726-730

Phillips MH, Stelzer KJ, Griffin TW, Mayerberg MR, Winn HR (1994) Stereotactic radiosurgery: a review and comparison of methods: J Clin Oncol 12: 1085-1099

Plowman PN (1997a) Stereotactical radiotherapy for arteriovenous malformations. Br J Neurosurg 11: 592

Plowman PN (1997b) Skeletal haemangiomatosis presenting with spinal cord compression- post-operative management of progressive disease. Br J Radiol 70: 429-431

Plowman PN, Harnett AN (1988) Radiotherapy in benign orbital disease 1. Complicated ocular angiomas. Br J Ophthalmol 72: 266-288

Plowman PN, Hungerford JL (1997) Radiotherapy for ocular angioma. Br J Ophthalmol 81: 258-259

Poulsen MG (1987) Arteriovenous malformations - a summary of 6 cases treated with radiation therapy. Int J Radiat Oncol Biol Phys 13: 1553-1557

Powell S, Peters N, Harmer C (1992) Chemodectoma of the head and neck: results of treatment in 84 patients. Int J Radiat Biol Phys 22(5): 919-24

Raco A, Ciapetta P, Artico M, Salvati M, Guidetti G, Guglielmo G (1990) Vertebral hemangiomas with cord compression: the role of embolisation in five cases. Surg Neurol 34: 164-168

Rogers LR, Morris HH, Lupica K (1993) Effect of cranial irradiation on seizure frequency in adults with low grade astrocytoma and medically intractable epilepsy. Neurology 453: 1599-1601

Roman G, Fisher M, Perl DP, Poser CM (1978) Neurological manifestations of hereditary haemorrhagic telangiectasia (Rendu - Osler - Weber disease): report of 2 cases and review of the literature. Ann Neurol 4: 130-144

Rossi GF, Scerrati M, Rosselli R (1985) Epileptic cerebral low grade tumours. Effect of interstitial stereotactic irradiation on seizures. Appl Neurophysiol 48: 127-132

Rotman M, John M, Stowe S, Inamdar S (1980) Radiation treatment of pediatric hepatic hemangiomatosis and co-existing heart failure. New Eng J Med 302: 852

Rubin P, Casaret GW (1968) Clinical radiation pathology. WB Saunders Company, Philadelphia pp 471-517

Saunders WM, Winston KR, Siddon RL et al. (1988) Radiosurgery for arteriovenous malformations of the brain using a standard linear accelerator: rationale and technique. Int J Radiat Oncol 15: 441-447

Scamoni C, Dario A, Basile L (1997) The association of cavernous and venous angioma. Case report and review of the literature. Br J Neurosurg 11: 346-349

Schild SE, Foote RL, Buskirk SJ, Robinew JS, Bock FF, Cupps RE, Earle JD (1992) Results of radiotherapy for chemodectomas. Mayo Clin Proc 67(6): 537-40

Schilling et al. (1997) Radiotherapy for choroidal haemangioma. Br J Ophthalmol 81: 267

Schipper J (1983) An accurate and simple method for megavoltage irradiation of retinoblastoma. Radiother Oncol 1: 31-41

Schlegel W, Pastyr O, Kubesch R et al. (1997) A computer controlled micro-multileaf collimator for stereotactic conformal radiotherapy. Proceedings of the XIIth ICCR meeting, Salt Lake City, Utah, May 1997

Sebag-Montefiore DSM, Biggs D, Dean E, Darlison R, Doughty D, Plowman PN (1994) Inoperable paediatric cerebral angiomas successfully treated by sterotactic radiotherapy. Proc Am Soc Clin Oncol 13: Abstr 1445

Sebag-Montefiore DJ, Doughty D, Biggs D, Plowman PN (1995) Stereotactic multiple arc radiotherapy 1. Vascular malformations of the brain: an analysis of the first 108 patients. J Neurosurg 9: 441-452

Simard JM, Grcia-Bengochea F, Ballinger WE, Mickle JP, Quisling RG (1986) Cavernous angioma: a review of 126 collected and 12 new clinical cases. Neurosurgery 18: 162-172

Skolyszewski J, Korzeniowski S, Pszon J (1991) Results of radiotherapy in chemodectoma of the temporal bone. Acta Oncol 30(7): 847-9

Springate SC, Haraf D, Weichselbaum RR (1991) Temporal bone chemodectomas - comparing surgery and radiation therapy. Oncology (Huntingt) 5(4): 131-7; discussion 140, 143

Steiner L, Lindquist C, Adler JR (1992) Clinical outcome of radiosurgery for cerebral arteriovenous malformations. J Neurosurg 77: 1-8

Steiner L, Lindquist C, Karlsson B, Guo W, Steiner M (1994) Gamma knife radiosurgery in cerebral vascular malformations. In: Pasqualin A, Da Pian R (eds) New trends in management of cerebrovascular malformations. Springer, Vienna, pp 473-485

Steinberg GK, Fabrikant JI, Marks MP et al. (1990) Stereotactic heavy charged particle Bragg-peak radiation for intracranial arteriovenous malformations. New Engl J Med 323: 96-101

Strandquist M (1939) Radium treatment of cutaneous of cutaneous haemangiomas using surface application of radium tubes in glass capsules. Acta Radiol 20: 185-211

Sutcliffe JC, Forster DMC, Walton L, Dias PS, Kennedy AA (1992) Untoward clinical effects after stereotactic radiosurgery for intracranial arteriovenous malformations. Br J Neurosurg 6: 177-185

Tagle P, Huette I, Mendez J, Del Villar S (1986) Intracranial cavernous angioma: presentation and management. J Neurosurg 64: 720-723

Thomson ES, Gill SS, Doughty D (1990) Stereotactic multiple arc radiotherapy. Br J Radiol 63: 745-751

Trott K (1991) Cardiovascular system morbidity of radiotherapy. In: Plowman PN, McElwain T, Meadows A (eds) Complications of cancer management. Butterworth-Heinemann, Oxford, pp 177-183

Wakai S, Ueda Y, Inoh S, Nagi M (1985) Angiographically occult angiomas. A report of 13 cases with analysis of the cases documented in the literature. Neurosurgery 17: 549-556

White RI, Lynch-Nyan A, Terry P (1988) Pulmonary arteriovenous malformations: techniques and long term outcome of embolotherapy. Radiology 169: 663-669

Willinsky RA, Lasjaunias P, Terbrugge K, Burrows P (1990) Multiple cerebral arteriovenous malformations (AVM): review of our experience of 203 patients with cerebral vascular malformations. Neuradiology 32: 207-210

Wilms G, Bleus E, Demaerel P et al. (1994) Simultaneous occurrence of developmental anomalies and cavernous angiomas. Am J Neuroradiol 15: 1247-1254

Yasargil MG (1988) Microneurosurgery. Volume 111b. AVM of the brain, clinical considerations, general and special operative techniques, surgical results, unoperated cases and venous angiomas, neuranaesthesia. Georg Thieme Verlag, New York, pp 418-435

Zografos L, Bercher L, Chamot L, Gailloud C, Raimondi S, Egger E (1996) Cobalt-60 treatment of choroidal angiomas. Am J Ophthalmol 121: 190-199

Index

A

Access, vascular *see* Vascular access
Adhesives 24-5, 34-7, 87-8
Amytal *see* Sodium amytal
Anatomy (spinal region) 97-9
Aneurysmal bone cyst 100
Aneurysms
  arterial 152
  cavernous 65-70
  cerebral *see* Intracranial aneurysms
  ectatic 41
  fusiform 5-6, 41
  giant 3, 29, 41, 46, 54
  infective (mycotic) 6-7
  intracranial *see* Intracranial aneurysms
  nidal (false) 80, 85
  non-saccular 5-7
  paraclinoid 65-6, 68
  saccular ("berry") 1-5, 39
  surgery indications 3-5
  surgical/endovascular combined treatment 13
  traumatic 6
  wide-necked 32-3, 41, 66, 69
Angioarchitecture 80, 83, 86
Angiographically occult vascular malformations (AOVM) 150-1
Angiography
  equipment 20
  preoperative 36
Angiomas
  cavernous 141, 142, 150
  familial incidence 142-3
  intracranial, radiosurgery 143-9
  radiation therapy history and rationale 139-43
  venous 12, 152
Angioplasty notes (carotid and vertebral artery) 110-16
AOVM *see* Angiographically occult vascular malformations
Apnoea 121
Arterial
  aneurysms 152
  embolisation (DAVMs) 59-61
  stents 108, 109
Arteriovenous fistulae (AVF) 36
  dural (DAVF) 57-61, 151-2
  spinal (SDAVF) 100-2
Arteriovenous malformations (AVM)
  cerebral 73-94, 120-2, 123-5

  childhood 10
  classification 75-7
  costs of treatments 94
  decision making 91-4
  dural (DAVM) 10-11, 57-61, 121
  embolisation complications 88-90
  embolisation techniques 19-27, 33-7, 83-6
  endovascular treatment 33-7, 86-90
  familial incidence 142-3
  grading (Spetzler and Martin) 33, 75-6, 81, 93, 124
  haemodynamics measurement 130-3
  haemorrhage risk
    factors 78-81
    table (Kondiziolka et al.) 92
  haemorrhaging and early treatment 90-1
  incidence 73
  monitoring
    neurological 119-34
    neurophysiological 123-6, 130-3
  morbidity and mortality 7-13, 77-8, 81-2
  multiple 75
  natural history 7-13, 77-8
  pregnancy 9-10
  radiation therapy 139-52
  radiosurgery 82-3, 85-6, 88, 93, 143-9
  seizures 80, 91, 146-7
  spinal cord 102-3, 122-3, 126
  surgery 81-6
  surgical/endovascular combined treatment 13-14
  treatment, special situations 90-1
Asymptomatic carotid stenosis 112
Atherosclerotic disease, carotid and vertebral artery, endovascular treatment 105-16
AVM *see* Arteriovenous malformations

B

Balloon occlusion 25, 26, 27-8, 66-9
  carotid artery 126-30
Basilar artery stenosis 114-15
"Berry" aneurysms *see* Saccular aneurysms
Biplanar digital fluoroscopy 20
Brachytherapy 142

C

Carotid artery occlusion, test balloon 126-30
Carotid cavernous fistulae (CCF) 61-5, 151-2
Carotid compression 59

Carotid PTA 110-13
Carotid stenosis, asymptomatic 112
Carotid territory, external (neurological monitoring) 122
Carotid and vertebral artery atherosclerotic disease, endovascular treatment 105-16
Carotid and Vertebral Artery Transluminal Angioplasty Study (CAVATAS) 111
Catheters 20-4, 83, 84
  cerebral protection 107
CAVATAS *see* Carotid and Vertebral Artery Transluminal Angioplasty Study
Cavernous aneurysms 65-70
Cavernous angiomas 141, 142, 150
Cavernous haemangiomas 11-12
Cavernous sinus lesions 57-70
CCF *see* Carotid cavernous fistulae
Cerebral aneurysms *see* Intracranial aneurysms
Cerebral arteriovenous malformations 73-94, 120-2
  neurophysiological monitoring 123-5
Cerebral protection catheters 107
Cerebrovascular PTA 105-16
Childhood AVMs 10
Classification of AVMs 75-7
  see also Spetzler and Martin AVM grading
Coaxial system *see* guiding catheters
Coil
  and catheter selection 49
  stretching (complication) 50
  types 24-5, 28-33
  see also Guglielmi detachable coil
Coiling and remodelling, cavernous aneurysms 69
CT *see* Xenon computed tomography (CT) scanning test
CT, *see also* Single photon emission computed tomography (SPECT)

D
DAVF *see* Dural arteriovenous fistulae
DAVM *see* Dural arteriovenous malformations
Delayed Ischaemic Deficit (DID) 51
Detachable microcoils 24-5, 28-33
  see also Guglielmi detachable coil
Detachable silicone balloons (DSB) 25, 26, 27-8, 63-4
Droperidol 125, 126
DSB *see* Detachable silicone balloons
Dural arteriovenous fistulae (DAVF) 57-61, 151-2
  spinal (SDAVF) 100-2
Dural arteriovenous malformations (DAVM) 10-11, 57-61, 121
  cavernous sinus 57-61

E
ECST *see* European Carotid Surgery Trial
Ectatic aneurysms 41
Electroencaphologram (EEG), (monitoring) 123-5, 130

Embolic agents 24-5
  see also Adhesives; Detachable microcoils; Detachable silicone balloons
Embolisation
  AVMs
    complications 88-90
    indications 84-5
    practical considerations 83-5
    and surgery 85-6
    techniques 19-27, 33-7, 83-6
  cerebral aneurysms 27-33
  spinal vascular abnormalities 99
Endosaccular occlusion of aneurysms 28-33
  complications 49-51
Endosaccular packing 45-54
Endovascular treatment
  arteriovenous malformations 33-7, 86-90
  carotid and vertebral artery atherosclerotic disease 105-16
  cerebral aneurysms 27-33
  intracranial aneurysms: Oxford experience 39-54
  neurological monitoring 119-34
  selection criteria 45-8
  spinal vascular abnormalities 97-103
Endovascular/surgical combined treatment (AVMs) 13-14
Epilepsy 80, 91, 146-7
Ethibloc adhesive 88
Ethylene vinyl alcohol copolymer (EVAL) 25
European Carotid Surgery Trial (ECST) 105
EVAL *see* Ethylene vinyl alcohol copolymer

F
Fentanyl 126
Fistulae
  arteriovenous (AVF) 36
  carotid cavernous (CCF) 61-5, 151-2
  dural arteriovenous (DAVF) 57-61, 151-2
  Spinal Dural Arteriovenous (SDAVF) 100-2
Flow-guided microcatheters 22-4, 84
Fusiform aneurysms 5-6, 41

G
Gamma knife 82, 143-6, 152
GDC *see* Guglielmi detachable coil
Giant aneurysms 3, 29, 41, 46, 54
Glomus jugulare tumours 152
Glue *see* Adhesives
Guglielmi detachable coil (GDC) 5, 24, 28-9, 30-2, 39, 44, 45
Guidewires, microcatheters 24
Guiding catheters 20, 21, 83

H
H/H/H (Triple H) therapy 51
Haemangiomas
  cavernous 11-12
  "strawberry" (capillary) 141
Haemodynamic and embolic consequences (after PTA) 112
Haemodynamics, AVM, (measurement) 130-3

Index

Haemorrhage
  AVM risk factors 78–81, 92
  and early AVM treatment 90–1
  see also Subarachnoid haemorrhage (SAH)
Haemostatic Valve and Flush 83–4
Heavy charged particle radiotherapy 144, 148–9
Helium radiotherapy 144, 148–9
Hippel-Lindau, Von, syndrome 141, 143
Histoacryl blue (NBCA monomer) 25, 34–7, 88
Hunt & Hess (HH) clinical grading 48
Hydrocephalus 51

I
IDC *see* Interlocking detachable coil
Infective (mycotic) aneurysms 6–7
Interlocking detachable coil (IDC) 28, 31
Interventional neuroradiology 82–3, 88
  embolisation techniques
    AVMs 19–27, 33–7, 83–6
    cerebral aneurysms 27–33
  neurophysiological monitoring 123–6, 130–3
Intra-aneurysmal clotting 47–8
Intracranial aneurysms
  endovascular treatment: Oxford experience 39–54
  morbidity and mortality 1–7
    procedural 52–4
  natural history 1–7
  surgical/endovascular treatment combined 13–14
  therapeutic options 27–33
Intracranial angiomas, radiosurgery 143–9
Ischaemic complications 50

K
Kondiziolka et al., AVM haemorrhage risk table 92

L
Leptomeningeal venous drainage 10–11, 57
Lidocaine 122, 123
Linear-accelerator-based radiosurgery 144, 146, 147

M
McCormick AVM classification (morphological) 75
Mayo Clinic 152
Mechanical detachable (coil) system (MDS) 25, 28, 31, 39
Medullary venous angiomas *see* Venous angiomas
Methohexitone 121
Microcatheters 20–4, 84
Microcoils
  detachable 24–5, 28–33
  see also Guglielmi detachable coil (GDC)
Monitoring
  electroencephalogram (EEG) 123–5, 130
  jugular bulb oxygen saturation 132–3
  neurological 119–34
  neurophysiological 123–6, 130–3

Morbidity and mortality
  AVMs 7–13, 77–8
  surgical 81–2
  intracranial aneurysms 1–7
  procedural 52–4

N
NASCET *see* North American Symptomatic Carotid Endarterectomy Trial
Natural history
  AVMs 7–13, 77–8
  intracranial aneurysms 1–7
NBCA monomer (adhesive) 25, 34–7, 88
Neurological monitoring 119–34
Neurophysiological monitoring 123–6, 130–3
Nidal (false) aneurysms 80, 85
Non-saccular intracranial aneurysms 5–7
North American Symptomatic Carotid Endarterectomy Trial (NASCET) 105

O
Occlusion
  aneurysms, endosaccular 28–33, 49–51
  balloon 25, 26, 27–8, 66–9
  carotid artery 126–30
  parent artery (PA) 27–8, 40–4
Ophthalmoplegia 66
Osler-Weber-Rendu syndrome 75, 142

P
Paraclinoid aneurysms 65–6, 68
Parent Artery (PA) occlusion 27–8, 40–4
Pentobarbitone 123
Percutaneous transfemoral endovascular treatment 14
Percutaneous transluminal angioplasty (PTA) 105–16
Pharmacological testing, provocative (neurological monitoring) 120–6
Pregnancy and arteriovenous malformations (AVMs) 9–10
Provocative pharmacological testing (neurological monitoring) 120–6
PTA *see* Percutaneous transluminal angioplasty

R
Radiation therapy
  angiomas, history and rationale 139–43
  and vascular malformations 139–52
Radiosurgery
  AVM 82–3, 85–6, 88, 93
  intracranial angiomas/AVMs 143–9
rCBF measurement 127–9
Recklinghausen, Von, disease 74
Rolandic fissure 80
Ruptured saccular aneurysms 1–2, 3–4

S
Saccular ("berry") aneurysms 1–5, 39
SAFE *see* Superselective anaesthesia functional examination
SAH *see* Subarachnoid haemorrhage

SDAVF *see* Spinal Dural Arteriovenous Fistulae
Seizures   80, 91, 146–7
Single photon emission computed tomography (SPECT)   127, 128–9
Sinus lesions, cavernous   57–70
Skeletal haemangiomatosis syndrome   143
Sodium amytal   86, 120–1, 122, 123
Somatosensory evoked potentials (SSEPs)   123, 125, 126, 130
SPECT *see* Single photon emission computed tomography
Spetzler and Martin AVM grading   33, 75–6, 81, 93, 124
Spinal anatomy   97–9
Spinal cord
  arteriovenous malformations (AVM)   102–3
  neurological monitoring   122–3, 126
Spinal Dural Arteriovenous Fistulae (SDAVF)   100–2
Spinal vascular abnormalities
  anatomy   97–9
  endovascular treatment   97–103
SSEPs *see* Somatosensory evoked potentials
Stents, arterial   108, 109
Stereotactic radiosurgery *see* Radiosurgery
"Strawberry" (capillary) haemangioma   141
Sturge-Weber syndrome   142, 143
Subarachnoid haemorrhage (SAH)   40, 42, 48
  coil/catheter induced   49–50
Subglottic angiomas   141
Superselective anaesthesia functional examination (SAFE)   120–1, 124
Surgery
  aneurysms   3–5
    early attempts   19–20
  AVMs   81–6
  carotid and vertebral artery atherosclerotic disease, disadvantages   105–6
Surgical/endovascular combined treatment   13–14

T
TCD *see* Transcranial Doppler ultrasonography
Thiopentone   121
TLA *see* Transluminal balloon angioplasty
Toronto Vascular Malformation Study Group   12
Transcranial Doppler ultrasonography (TCD)   110, 127, 129–33
Transluminal balloon angioplasty (TLA)   51
Transvenous approach (DAVFs)   61
Traumatic aneurysms   6
Triple H (H/H/H) therapy   51

U
Unruptured saccular aneurysms   2–3, 4–5

V
Vascular access   26–7, 29–32, 45
Vascular malformations
  natural history   7–13, 77–8
  see also Arteriovascular malformations (AVM)
Vasospasm   51
Venous angiomas   12, 152
Venous drainage classification (DAVM/F)   57
Vertebral artery and carotid atherosclerotic disease, endovascular treatment   105–16
Vertebral artery stenosis   114
Von Hippel-Lindau syndrome   141, 143
Von Recklinghausen disease   74

W
Wide-necked aneurysms   32–3, 41, 66, 69
World Federation of Neurological Surgeons (WFNS) clinical grading   48
Wyburn-Mason syndrome   75

X
Xenon computed tomography (CT) scanning test   67, 127–9

Made in the USA
Columbia, SC
06 June 2025